Table of Contents

Chapter One

- Standard I
- Standard II
- Standard III
- Standard IV
- Standard VI
- Standard VI
- Standard VII
- Standard VIII

I0470893

Chapter Two

- Legal and Ethical Aspects of Nursing
- Ethical Concepts That Apply to Nursing Practice
- Nursing Code (ANA)
- Legal Concepts That Apply to Nursing Practice
- Good Samaritan Doctrine
- Legal Responsibilities of the Nurse

Chapter Three

- Managing Client Care Safety
- Application of Maslow's Hierarchy in Health Care
- Safety and Security Needs
- Assignment Methods for Delivery of Care

Chapter Four

- Fire Safety and Preparedness Practices
- Prevention is everyone's responsibility
- Restraints
- Body Mechanics
- Transfer and Movement Principles and Techniques

Chapter Five

- Positions
- Nursing Abbreviations
- NCLEX Prep 265 Question Quizz
- Coordinate Care Quizz
- Infection Control Quizz
- Delegation of Care Quizz
- Priority of Care Quizz
- Nursing Care Management Quizz
- References and Source of Information

Nursing Care Management

Nurses must frequently apply various management principles while caring for their clients in various health care settings. This unit has been crafted to clarify these issues. It begins with a comprehensive view of nursing practice standards as well as legal and ethical aspects of nursing. Client care management issues such as determining priorities, working with the health care team, making assignments, and coordinating client care as the client progresses from admission through discharge have been described along with valuable principles to facilitate the nurse's application of this information.

Safety considerations regarding fire, electricity, equipment, and the use of physical restraints have been incorporated. This unit also includes selected principals and interventions related to specific aspects of care such as body mechanics, transfer techniques, positioning, application of cold and heat, asepsis, and the care of clients who develop or are at risk for pressure ulcers.

STANDARDS OF NURSING PRACTICE

Nursing practice is a direct service that is goal directed and adaptable to the needs of the individual, family, and community during health and illness.

Professional practitioners of nursing bear primary responsibility and accountability for the nursing care clients receive.

The purpose of the Standards of Nursing Practice is to fulfill the profession's obligation to provide and improve this practice. The Standards focus on practice.

They provide a means for determining the quality of nursing a client receives regardless of whether such services are provided solely by a professional nurse or by a professional nurse and nonprofessional assistants.

The Standards are stated according to a systematic approach to nursing practice: the assessment of the client's status, the plan of nursing actions, the implementation of the plan, and the evaluation. These specific divisions are not intended to imply that practice consists of a series of discrete steps, taken in strict sequence, beginning with assessment and ending with evaluation.

The processes described are used concurrently and recurrently. Assessment, for example, frequently continues during implementation; similarly, evaluation dictates reassessment and re-planning.

These Standards for Nursing Practice apply to nursing practice in any setting. Nursing practice in all settings must possess the characteristics identified by these Standards if clients are to receive a high quality of nursing care. Each Standard is followed by a rationale and assessment factors. Assessment factors are to be used in determining achievement of the standard.

Chapter One

STANDARDS FOR NURSING CARE

Nurses must frequently apply various management principles while caring for their clients in various health care settings. This unit has been crafted to clarify these issues. It begins with a comprehensive view of nursing practice standards as well as legal and ethical aspects of nursing.

Client care management issues such as determining priorities, working with the health care team, making assignments, and coordinating client care as the client progresses from admission through discharge have been described along with valuable principles to facilitate the nurse's application of this information.

Safety considerations regarding fire, electricity, equipment, and the use of physical restraints have been incorporated. Also includes interventions related to specific aspects of care such as body mechanics, transfer techniques, positioning, application of cold and heat, asepsis, and the care of clients who develop or are at risk for pressure ulcers.

STANDARD I –Assessment and Data Collection

The collection of data about the health status of the client is systematic and continuous. The data are accessible, communicated, and recorded.

Rationale

Comprehensive care requires complete and ongoing collection of data about the client. All health status data about the client must be available for all members of the health care team.

Assessment Factors

Health status data include:

- Growth and development
- Biophysical status
- Emotional status
- Cultural, religious, socioeconomic background
- Performance of activities of daily living
- Patterns of coping
- Interaction patterns
- Client's perception of and satisfaction with his health status
- Client health goals
- Environment (physical, social, emotional, ecological)
- Available and accessible human and material resources

Data are collected from:

1. Client
2. Health care personnel
3. Individuals within the immediate environment and/or the community
4. Data are obtained by:
5. Interview
6. Examination
7. Observation
8. Reading records, reports, etc.
9. There is a format for the collection of data that:
10. Provides for a systematic collection of data
11. Facilitates the completeness of data collection
12. Continuous collection of data is evident by:
13. Frequent updating
14. Recording of changes in health status

The data are:

- Accessible on the client records
- Retrievable from record-keeping systems
- Confidential when appropriate

STANDARD II – Diagnoses

Nursing diagnoses are derived from health status data obtained from the patient's assessment; thus such assessment providing the basis for planning, implementing and evaluation of the health status and recovery of the patient in a safe and effective manner, the ultimate goal of nursing intervention.

Rationale
The health status of the client is the basis for determining the nursing care needs. The data are analyzed and compared to norms whenever possible throughout the nursing porcess to effecgively and safely intervene for the patient's health and recovery.

Assessment Factors
The client's health status is compared to the norm in order to determine if there is a deviation from the norm and the degree and direction of deviation. The client's capabilities and limitations are identified. The nursing diagnoses are related to and congruent with the diagnoses of all other professionals caring for the client.

STANDARD III –Planning and Implementing

The plan of nursing care includes goals derived from the nursing diagnosis. A course for planning, implementation and evaluation of intervention derives directly from a diagnosis. At this point at the nursing process the health history of the patient is analyzed to his/her current health status and compared to normal health values and used as guidelines for planning and implementing the intervention intended to reestablish the client's health to normal values.

Rationale

The determination of the results to be achieved is an essential part of planning care. Other diagnosis derived nursing interventions are implementing treatment and evaluation of the sam as the recovery of the client's needs is reached.

Assessment Factors

- Goals are mutually set with the client and pertinent others.
- They are congruent with other planned therapies.
- They are stated in realistic and measurable terms.
- They are assigned a time period for achievement.
- Goals are established to maximize functional capabilities

Goals must be congruent with:

- Growth and development
- Biophysical status
- Behavioral patterns
- Human and material resources

STANDARD IV – Care Priroritty and Approach

The plan of nursing care includes priorities and the prescribed nursing approaches or measures to achieve the goals derived from the nursing diagnoses.

Rationale

Nursing actions are planned to promote, maintain, and restore the client's well being. The steps are planned to achieve the final nursing intervention goal: recover of the client's health status within the shortest time possible in a safely and effectively approach.

Assessment Factors –Physiological and Psychological Measures

Physiological measures are planned to manage (prevent or control) specific client problems and are related to the nursing diagnoses and goals of care, e.g., ADL, use of self-help devices, while Psychosocial measures are specific to the client's nursing care problem and to the nursing care goals, e.g., the social-integrity of the client as a way to incorporate techniques to control aggression, motivation, etc addding to the care of the client.

Teaching-learning principles are incorporated as well into the plan of care and objectives for learning stated in behavioral terms, e.g., specification of content for learner's level, reinforcement, readiness, etc. Approaches are planned to provide for a therapeutic environment.

Physical environmental factors are used to influence the therapeutic environment, e.g., control of noise, control of temperature, light, etc. while psychosocial measures are used to structure the environment for therapeutic ends, e.g., paternal participation in all phases of the maternity experience, while group behaviors are used to structure interaction and influence the therapeutic environment, e.g., conformity, ethos, territorial rights, locomotion, aimed at psychosocial integrity of the client.

Approaches to Planning

The plan includes an ordered sequence of nursing actions. Nursing approaches are planned on the basis of current scientific knowledge.

Approaches are specified for orientation of the client to:

- New roles and relationships
- Relevant health (human and material) resources
- Modifications in plan of nursing care
- Relationship of modifications in nursing care plan to the total care plan

The plan of nursing care includes the utilization of available and appropriate resources:

- Human resources
- Other health personnel
- Material resources
- Community

STANDARD V – Health Promotion

Nursing actions provide for client participation in health promotion, maintenance, and restoration of halth to nomal standards.

Rationale

The client and family are continually involved in nursing care as part of the physical and psychosocial recovery of the client.

Assessment Factors

The client and family are kept informed about:
- Current health status
- Changes in health status
- Total health care plan
- Nursing care plan
- Roles of health care personnel
- Health care resources

The client and family are provided with the information needed to make decisions and choices about promoting, maintaining, and restoring health. Seeking and utilizing appropriate health care personnel and maintaining and using health care resources

STANDARD VI

Nursing actions assist the client to maximize his health capabilities. Thoroughtout the entire nursing intervention, the nurse is an uncompromised surrogate for the client's health needs.

Rationale

Nursing actions are designed to promote, maintain, and restore health within the strictest parameters of safe and effective intervention.

Assessment Factors

Nursing actions:

- Are consistent with the plan of care.
- Are based on scientific principles.
- Are individualized to the specific situation.
- Are used to provide a safe and therapeutic environment.
- Employ teaching-learning opportunities for the client.
- Include utilization of appropriate resources.

Nursing actions are directed by the client's physical, physiological, psychological, and social behavior associated with the client's health condition, including:

- Ingestion of food, fluid, and nutrients
- Elimination of body wastes and excesses in fluid
- Locomotion and exercise
- Regulatory mechanisms--body heat, metabolism
- Relating to others
- Self-actualization

STANDARD VII

The client's progress or lack of progress toward goal achievement is determined by the client and the nurse.

Rationale

The quality of nursing care depends upon comprehensive measure and intelligent determination of nursing's impact upon the health status of the client. The client is an essential part of this determination.

Assessment Factors

Current data about the client are used to measure his progress toward goal achievement. Nursing actions are analyzed for their effectiveness in the goal achievement of the client. The client evaluates nursing actions and goal achievement. Provision is made for nursing follow-up of a particular client to determine the long-term effects of nursing care.

STANDARD VIII

The client's progress or lack of progress toward goal achievement directs reassessment, reordering of priorities, new goal setting, and revision of the plan of nursing care.

Rationale

The nursing process remains the same, but the input of new information may dictate new or revised approaches.

Assessment Factors

Reassessment is directed by goal achievement or lack of goal achievement. New priorities and goals are determined and additional nursing approaches are prescribed appropriately. New nursing actions are accurately and appropriately initiated.

Chapter Two

Legal and Ethical Aspects of Nursing

OVERVIEW

Legal responsibilities are regulated by State nurse-practice acts and may vary from State to State. It is important for nurses to recognize that nursing practice is guided by legal restrictions and professional obligations.

In addition, general standards for the practice of nursing have been developed and published by the American Nurses' Association, which has also developed a Code of Ethics.

Nurses need to be aware of these standards, as well as legal and ethical concepts and principles, since nurses are accountable for their actions in all these areas in their professional role; this undertanding is specially helpful to international educated nurses.

Ethical Concepts That Apply to Nursing Practice

Ethics: are pre-established rules and principles that guide nursing decisions or conduct in terms of the rightness/wrongness of that decision or action.

Morals: personally held beliefs, opinions, and attitudes that guide our actions.

Values: appraisal of what is "good."

Dilemmas may occur when different values conflict. Religious values may enter in conflict with nursing practices.

Example: client's right to refuse treatment on religous tenets may be in conflict with nurse's obligation to benefit client and to carry out treatment.

Ethical Dilemma

Is a problem in making a decision because there is no clearly correct or right choice. This may result in having to choose an action that violates one principle or value in order to promote another. Amongst these delimmas are:

-Autonomy: an individual right to make his/her own decision regarding treatment and care.
-Paternalism: another person makes decisions about what's right/best for individual.
-Beneficence: promoting good or doing no harm to another.
-Right to know: right to knowledge necessary or helpful in making an informed decision.
-Principle of double effect: promoting good may involve some expected harm.
-Distributive justice: allocation of goods/services and how or to whom they are distributed.
-Equality: everyone receives the same.
-Need: greater services go to those with greater needs (e.g., critically ill client receives more intensive nursing care).
-Merit: services go to more deserving (used as a criterion for transplant recipients).

CODE FOR NURSES (ANA, 1985)

The nurse provides services with respect for human dignity and the uniqueness of the client, unrestricted by considerations of social or economic status, personal attributes, or the nature of health problems. The nurse safeguards the client's right to privacy by judiciously protecting information of a confidential nature.

The nurse acts to safeguard the client and the public when health care and safety are affected by the incompetent, unethical, or illegal practice of any person.

The nurse assumes responsibility and accountability for individual nursing judgments and actions.

(1)   The nurse maintains competence in nursing.

(2)   The nurse exercises informed judgment and uses individual competence and qualifications as criteria in seeking consultation, accepting responsibilities, and delegating nursing activities to others.

(3)   The nurse participates in activities that contribute to the ongoing development of the profession's body of knowledge.

(4)   The nurse participates in the profession's efforts to implement and improve standards of nursing.

(5)   The nurse participates in the profession's efforts to establish and maintain conditions of employment conducive to high-quality nursing care.

(6)   The nurse participates in the profession's efforts to protect the public from misinformation and misrepresentation and to maintain the integrity of nursing.

(7)   The nurse collaborates with members of the health professions and other citizens in promoting community and national efforts to meet the health needs of the public.

Legal Concepts That Apply to Nursing Practice

Standards: identify the minimal knowledge and conduct expected from a professional practitioner. Standards are applied as they relate to a practitioner's experience and educational preparation.

For example, any nurse would be expected to be certain that an ordered medication was being given to the correct client.

However, more complex nursing actions, such as respirator monitoring, would require supervised experience and/or continuing education.

Definitions

Negligence: lack of reasonable conduct or care. Omitting an action expected of a prudent person in a particular circumstance is considered negligence, as is committing an action that a prudent person would not.

Malpractice: professional negligence, misconduct, or unreasonable lack of skill resulting in injury or loss to the recipient of the professional services.
Competence: ability or qualification to make informed decisions.

Informed consent: agreement to the performance of a procedure/treatment based on knowledge of facts, risks, and alternatives.

Simple: having capacity to give consent for the treatment or procedure.

Valid: having capacity to give consent and also demonstrating an understanding of the nature of the treatment, expected effects, possible side effects, and alternatives to treatment.

Assault: unjustifiable threat or attempt to touch or injure another.

Battery: unlawful touching or injury to another.

Crime: act that is a violation of duty or breach of law, punishable by the state by fine or imprisonment.

Tort: a legal wrong committed against a person, his or her rights, or property; intentional, willfully committed without just cause (see Illustration 1). The person who commits a tort is liable for damages in a civil action. Negligence and malpractice are torts.

Victims of malpractice are entitled to receive monetary awards (damages) to compensate for their injury or loss.

Good Samaritan Doctrine

A rescuer is protected from liability when assisting in an emergency situation or rescuing a person from imminent and serious peril, if attempt is not reckless and person's condition is not made worse. The Good Samaritan doctrine is used by rescuers to avoid civil liability for injuries arising from their negligence.

Its purpose is to encourage emergency assistance by removing the threat of liability for damage done by the assistance. However, the assistance must be reasonable; a rescuer cannot benefit from the Good Samaritan doctrine if the assistance is reckless or grossly negligent.

Three key elements support a successful invocation of the Good Samaritan doctrine: (1) the care rendered was performed as the result of the emergency, (2) the initial emergency or injury was not caused by the person invoking the defense, and (3) the emergency care was not given in a grossly negligent or reckless manner.

Assume that a person has slipped on ice and broken a vertebra. The victim is unconscious, the accident has occurred in a desolate area, and the weather is dangerously cold.

A passerby finds the injured person and moves the person to warmth and safety, but in the process aggravates the spinal injury. In a civil suit by the victim seeking damages for the additional injury, the passerby may successfully defeat the claims under the Good Samaritan doctrine.

The Good Samaritan doctrine is also used as a defense by persons who act to prevent or contain property damage. Assume that a passerby notices a fire has started just outside a cabin in the wilderness. If the passerby breaks into the cabin to look for a fire extinguisher, the passerby will not be liable for damage resulting from the forced entry.

However, if the passerby runs down the cabin with a bulldozer to extinguish the fire, this will probably be considered grossly negligent or reckless, and the Good Samaritan doctrine will not provide protection from a civil suit for damages to the cabin.

A principle of **Tort Law** *that provides that a person who sees another individual in imminent and serious danger or peril cannot be charged with* **Negligence** *if that first person attempts to aid or rescue the injured party, provided the attempt is not made recklessly.*

Many states are content to follow the Good Samaritan doctrine through their Common Law or through similar previous cases.

Some states have general statutes mandating the doctrine.

Utah, for example, has a Good Samaritan act, which provides in part that [a] person who renders emergency care at or near the scene of, or during an emergency, gratuitously and in Good Faith, is not liable for any civil damages or penalties as a result of any act or omission by the person rendering the emergency care, unless the person is grossly negligent or caused the emergency. (Utah Code Ann. § 78-11-22).

Licensure Granted by states to Protect Public.

Purposes

- Standards for entry into practice
- Defines what licensed person can do (e.g., Nurse Practice Acts)
- License revocation/suspension
- Criteria vary in each state.
- Licensed nurses should be aware of their state's nurse practice act.
- Nurses who are disciplined in one state may also be disciplined in another state in which they hold a license.

Legal Concepts Related to Psychiatric-Mental Health Nursing

Voluntary commitment

The client consents to hospital admission. Client must be released when he or she no longer chooses to remain in the hospital. State laws govern how long a client must remain hospitalized prior to release. Client has the right to refuse treatment.

Involuntary commitment

The client is hospitalized without consent. Most states require that the client be mentally ill and be a danger to others/self (includes being unable to meet own basic needs such as eating or protection from injury). In most states the client who has been involuntarily committed may not refuse treatment.

Insanity: a legal term for mental illness where an individual cannot be held responsible for or does not understand the nature of his or her acts.

Insanity defenses: not guilty by reason of insanity.

M'Naghten rule ("right and wrong test"):

the accused is not legally responsible for an act if, at the time the act was committed, the person did not, because of mental defect or illness, know the nature of the act or that the act was wrong.

Irresistible impulse:

The accused, because of mental illness, did not have the will to resist an impulse to commit the act, even though able to differentiate between right and wrong. Individuals who commit crimes and successfully plead insanity defenses may be ordered to involuntary committed to psychiatric hospitals under civil commitment laws. There is presently a trend toward finding individuals insane and guilty.

Rights of Clients (Patients)

Rights that each state may grant to its residents committed to a psychiatric hospital.

- Right to receive treatment and not just be confined
- Right to the least restrictive care - locked/unlocked units, inpatient/outpatient.
- Right to individualized treatment plan and to
- Right to participation in development of plan
- Right to explanation of the treatment
- Right to confidentiality of records
- Right to visitors, mail, and use of telephone
- Right to refuse to participate in experimental treatments
- Right to freedom from seclusion or restraints
- Right to an explanation of rights and assertion of grievances
- Right to due process

Legal Responsibilities of the Nurse

- A nurse is expected to be responsible for his or her own acts
- Protect the rights and safety of patients
- Witness, but not obtain, informed consent for medical procedures
- Document and communicate information regarding client care and responses
- Refuse to carry out orders that the nurse knows/believes harmful to the client
- Perform acts allowed by that nurse's state nurse practice act
- Reveal client's confidential information only to appropriate persons
- Perform acts for which the nurse is qualified by either education or experience
- Witness a will (this is not a legal obligation, but the nurse may choose to do so)
- Restrain clients only in emergencies to prevent injury to self/others.
- Clients have the right to be free from unlawful restraint.

Chapter Three

Managing Client Care Safety

PRIORITIES OF CLIENT CARE

For One Client

Maslow's Hierarchy of Needs (1954)

Principles

An individual's needs are depicted in ascending levels on the hierarchy. Needs on one level must be (at least partially) met before one can focus on a higher-level need.

Levels of Maslow's Hierarchy

Physiologic/survival needs: basic human needs (e.g., oxygen, water, food, elimination, physical and mental rest, activity, and avoidance of pain)

Safety and Security Needs

- Protection from physical harm (e.g., mechanical, thermal, chemical, or infectious)

- Interpersonal, economic, and emotional security

- Affection or belonging needs

- Giving and receiving of affection

- Sense of belonging (e.g., including client/family in planning of care)

- Self-esteem/respect needs Feeling of self-worth Need for recognition Self-actualization.

Highest level: not reached by all

- Independence

- Feeling of achievement or competency

Application of Maslow's Hierarchy in Health Care

Client Care

Basic physiologic needs should take precedence over higher-level needs and on up the continuum accordingly. Professional nurse often delivers care at multiple levels simultaneously (e.g., while feeding a client, you position them to prevent aspiration and converse with them). Tool to guide decision making of priorities in emergencies and time management of care. Also applies to families, staff, and yourself

For Multiple Clients

Maslow's Hierarchy applies (e.g., more critically ill clients will require more care to meet their physiologic/survival needs)

- Organizing multiple client assignments

- Analyze and plan for entire shift.

- Develop a working plan so that priorities get accomplished and all clients receive optimal care.

- First consider schedules for nursing activities (e.g., meds, treatments, VS, mealtimes, client appointments, I&Os, etc.).

Then work in the nonscheduled activities that need to be accomplished to meet care plan goals (e.g., supporting family, teaching client, meeting with other departments about scheduling, writing care plan, discharge planning).

ASSIGNMENT METHODS FOR DELIVERY OF CARE

Principles

- RN is the decision maker/delegator

- Assesses each client.

- Determines appropriate plan of care.

- Assesses available staff and their job descriptions.

- Decides how to use human resources to accomplish care.

Typical levels of staff

Nursing Assistants

Least-skilled workers

Assign to majority of the "routine" procedures (e.g., baths, bed making, routine VS, etc.)

Licensed Practical Nurse (LPN)/Licensed Vocational Nurse (LVN)

LPN/LVN is the technical doer.

Assign to physical care of clients with more complex conditions, selected treatments, and perhaps some medications.

Registered Nurse (RN)

- Performs the most complex procedures (e.g., starting IVs, developing the plan of care, interpreting EKGs, correlating laboratory results with client status)
- Applies the nursing process for each client.
- Coordinates the medical plan with the nursing care plan
- Coordinates client activities
- Other departments

Health care workers

Community

- Performs client/family teaching
- Ensures documentation of care and outcomes
- Directs and supervises care given by LPNs and ancillary personnel
- Acts as a client advocate - Supporting, pleading, or arguing in favor of the client
- Client rights
- Facility policy
- Treatment/care issues
- Personnel issues

Admission of Client to Hospital

- Room assignment
- Check available data (e.g., diagnosis, age, pertinent history)
- Does client need to be close to nurses' station for optimal monitoring?
- Does client need isolation or special precautions?
- Who will be the client's roommate?

Consider the physical layout of available rooms and bathrooms. What would be best for the client based on his or her functional status? Perform a baseline admission assessment per facility procedure. Obtain needed equipment (e.g., urinal, denture cup, etc.).

Record on clothing record and explain/ document the disposition of valuables per facility policy.

- Orient to facility/policies (e.g., visiting hours, parking, telephone, chaplaincy services, TV, mealtimes, electrical equipment, etc.).

- Orient to unit (e.g., layout, lounges, smoking policy, activities, menu selection, medication times, straight vs. prn orders, mealtimes, unit personnel, etc.).

- Orient to room (e.g., roommate; bedside stand, table, and closet; call light,bathroom call system, bed operation, TV, telephone, etc.).

Caring for the Client Who Leaves the Unit

Coordinate scheduling to consider client's diagnosis, activity/test to be performed, and client's other therapeutic goals. Prepare client physically and psychologically as indicated. Consider the client's condition; medication, diet, and treatment regimes; as well as specific precautions and adjust the client's schedule as needed. Communicate pertinent information to other departments/personnel.

Discharge of Client from the Hospital

Discharge to home.

Begin discharge plan on admission. Teach client/significant other about disease process, needed precautions, restrictions, treatments, and medications. Assess and document knowledge of disease and home-care regimen and ability to perform safely. Make referrals as needed for added support and care (e.g., community/home health nurses, home health aide, community support groups, other disciplines, i.e., social worker, physical therapist, etc.). Arrange for client to obtain needed equipment/supplies (e.g., bedside commode, supplies, dressings, etc.).

Prescriptions Availability

Ensure that client has needed prescriptions. Provide written/audio educational materials at the level of the client's ability. Schedule or direct client to arrange for appropriate follow-up. Communicate with individuals/agency(ies) responsible for follow-up care. Discharge of Client to Long-term Care Facility Communicate with facility nursing staff

- Client's functional abilities and limitations

- Present medical regime and schedule

- Mental and behavioral status

- Family support/involvement

- Nursing care plan and response

- Existing advance directives

- Recent medication administration records

- History and Physical

- Pertinent diagnostic reports

- Other: requirements per insurance

Chapter Four

Safety

FIRE SAFETY/PREPAREDNESS PRACTICES

- Be aware of hazards and report immediately.
- Locate and remember
- Escape routes
- Fire drill procedures.
- Use of available equipment
- Fire escapes
- Fire doors
- Fire alarms
- Fire sprinkler controls
- Fire extinguishers and/or medical air
- Keep fire exits clear.
- Fire Safety
- Shut off valves for O2

Prevention is everyone's responsibility.

Three elements needed for a fire to start

- **Fuel--substance that will burn**
- **Heat--flame or spark**
- **Oxygen--room air contains 21% O.**

In the event of a fire

- **Move clients to safety if in immediate vicinity of fire**
- **Sound the alarm**
- **Close all windows and doors**

If selected clients need continuous O2 or medical air, attach to emergency provisions once they are removed from vicinity of fire. Shut off piped-in O2 and/or medical air. Follow institutional policy concerning announcing the fire and location and notifying fire company. Avoid use of elevators. Follow institutional evacuation plan as needed.

EQUIPMENT

Follow facility procedure when using various equipment. When unfamiliar equipment contact your staff development department or supervisor for information. Read available manufacturer's literature. Suspected malfunction 1) doesn't do its task consistently or correctly, 2) makes unusual noises, 3) gives off an unusual odor or extreme temperature)

- Don't try to repair.
- Replace it immediately.
- Contact maintenance so that it can be checked out safely and repaired.

RESTRAINTS

Physical restraints should be used only if necessary to prevent injury to the client or others.

Physicians Orders

Signed, dated, physician's order needs to be written specifying the form of restraint and a time limit for restraint use. At that time the client will be reevaluated for restraint need to determine if a less restrictive method is appropriate.

- Least restrictive form of restraint should be used

- Maintain functional abilities

- Decrease risk of complications

- Minimize behavioral reaction

Remove restraints for 10 min q2h for ROM, repositioning/ambulation, toileting, and preventative skin care. Document rationale for restraint, other measures tried in lieu of restraint (e.g., pillows, environmental modifications, etc.), client response, and preventative care.

INTERVENTIONS FOR SPECIFIC ASPECTS OF CARE

Body Mechanics

- Safe and efficient use of appropriate muscle groups to do the job
- Principles for the safe movement of clients
- Keep your back straight.
- Ensure a wide base of support (keep your feet separated).
- Bend from the hips and knees (not the waist).
- Use the major muscle groups (strongest).
- Use your body weight to help push or pull.
- Avoid twisting. (Pivot the whole body.)
- Hold heavy objects close to your body.
- Push or pull objects instead of lifting.
- Ask for help as needed.
- Synchronize efforts with client and other staff.
- Use turning or lifting sheets as needed.
- Use mechanical devices as needed.

Transfer and Movement Principles and Techniques

From bed to chair or wheelchair.

Identify client's strongest side. Place chair beside bed, on same side as client's strongest side, so it faces the foot of bed. Stabilize chair and lock wheels. Lower bed, lock wheels, and elevate head of bed. If assistance is needed:

Place one arm under client's shoulders. The other arm should be placed over and around the knees. Bring legs over the side of bed while raising the client's shoulders off of the bed. Dangle client and watch for signs of fainting or dizziness. (Stand in front of client for protection in case of balance problems.) paralyzed arm during transfer. (Use sling or clothing for support.)

Place client's feet flat on the floor. (If client has a weak leg, use your leg and foot to brace the weak foot and knee.) Face the client and grasp firmly by placing your arms under the arm pits. Have client lean forward so that your control of the client's upper body is stabilized.

Using a wide base of support and bending at your knees, coach the client to assist as much as possible by using verbal instruction and counting. Stand client (if weight bearing is permitted) by pivoting the feet, legs, and hips to a standing position. Continue the slow pivotal movement until client is positioned over chair. Lower client into chair.

Log Rolling

Performed when spinal column must be kept straight (post-injury or surgery). Two or more persons needed. Both staff should be on side opposite where client is to be turned.

- One staff places hands under client's head and shoulders.
- One staff places hands under client's hips and legs.
- Move client as a unit toward you.
- Cross arms over chest and place pillow between legs.
- Raise side rail.
- Both staff move to side of bed to which client is being turned.
- One staff should be positioned to keep client's shoulders and hips straight.
- One staff should be positioned to keep thighs and lower legs straight.
- At the same time the client is drawn toward both staff in a single unified motion.
- The client's head, spine and legs are kept in a straight position.
- Position with pillows for support and raise side rails.

Positioning of the Client

General principles

- Privacy/draping

- Universal precautions as needed

Knowledge of client's condition when moving client (e.g., paresis or paralysis of a limb; need to support joints or limbs in a specific manner;awareness of pressure points)

- Good posture and body alignment

Use of added supports as needed (e.g., pillows, wedge cushions, handrolls, foot boards, **etc.) Comfort--reduce pressure and strain on body parts**

Safety

Bed in a low position once repositioned Access to personal items and care (e.g., call bell, drinking water, tissues, telephone, etc.) Clients should change position fairly frequently (at least every 2 hours).

Chapter Five

Positions

Semi-Fowler's

Backrest elevated at 45° angle. Knees supported in slight flexion. Arms rest at sides

High Fowler's

Backrest elevated at 90° angle (right angle). Knees slightly flexed. Arms supported on pillows or bedside table. Allows for good chest expansion in clients with cardiac or respiratory problems

Supine (dorsal/horizontal recumbent)

Client lies on his back. Client's head and shoulders slightly elevated with pillow (modified per client condition, physician order or agency policy regarding spinal injury/ surgery or post spinal anesthesia) Small pillow under lumbar curvature. Prevent external rotation of legs with supports placed laterally to trocanters. Knees slightly flexed. Prevent footdrop with foot board, rolled pillow or high top sneakers (depends on persistence of client condition)

Prone

- Client lies on his abdomen.
- Head turned to one side on small pillow or on flat surface.
- Small pillow just below diaphragm to support lumbar curve, facilitate breathing, and decrease pressure on female breasts.
- Pillow under lower legs to reduce plantar flexion and flex knees.
- May be modified in amputees where flexion of hips and knees may be contraindicated.

Trendelenburg

Client lies on back with head lower than rest of body.
Enhances circulation to the heart and brain. Sometimes used when shock is present.

In emergencies, the entire lower bed may be elevated on "shock blocks."
May be used for prolapsed cord outside of the hospital.

Modified Trendelenburg

Client is positioned with legs elevated to an angle of approximately 20°, knees straight, trunk horizontal, and head slightly elevated. Used for persons in shock to improve cerebral circulation and venous return to the heart without compromising respiration. (Contraindicated when head injury is present.)

Lateral (side-lying)

Client lies on his side.
Pillow under head to prevent lateral neck flexion and fatigue. Both arms are slightly flexed in front of the body. Pillow under the upper arm and shoulder provides support and permits easier chest expansion. Pillow under upper leg and thigh prevents internal rotation and hip adduction. Rolled pillow behind client's back.

Sims' (semiprone)

Similar to lateral, but with weight supported on anterior aspects of the ilium, humerous, and clavicle. Used for vaginal and rectal exams, enema administration, and drainage of oral secretions from the unconscious client. Comfortable for the client in the last trimester of pregnancy. Client placed on side (left side for enema or rectal exam) with head turned to side on a pillow. Lower arm is extended behind the body. Upper arm flexed in front of body and supported by a pillow. Upper leg is sharply flexed over pillow with the lower leg slightly bent.

Knee-chest

Client first lies on abdomen with head turned to one side on apillow. Arms flexed on either side of head. Finally the client is assisted to flex and draw knees up to meet the chest. Difficult position to be maintained--do not leave client alone. Used for rectal and vaginal exams.

Dorsal lithotomy

Used for female pelvic exam. Have client void before assuming this position. Client lies on back with the knees well flexed and separated. Frequently stirrups are used. (Adjust for proper feet and lower leg support.) If prolonged use of stirrups, be alert to signs of clot formation in the pelvis and lower extremities.

Cold Application

Warm and cold applications provide healing and promote comfort to areas of the body that are injured or have an inflammatory process. It is important to understand the principles of warm and cold applications and use this knowledge to ably and safely apply the different methods of warm and cold treatment procedures. Client lies on top of one, or between two, cooling blankets. Blanket(s) are attached to a machine that circulate(s) coolant solution.

Follow agency policy/procedure for care of client treated with hypothermia blanket(s). Monitor VS (T, P, R, and BP) regularly and frequently. Attention to skin hygiene and protection with oil as required. Frequent repositioning and assessment of body surface areas. Observe for signs of tissue damage and frostbite (pale areas). Assist client in basic needs (e.g., hygiene, elimination, nutrition, etc.). Identify client temperature at which to cease the treatment (temperature may continue to drift downward). Monitor VS frequently until stable for 72 hours.

Alcohol or sponge bath (tepid solutions, 85°-100°F)

Alcohol bath--combination of alcohol and water (alcohol has a drying effect on skin--used less frequently). Alcohol increases heat loss by evaporation.

Sponge bath--cool or tepid (not cold) water.

Frequent and regular VS monitoring (T, P, R, and BP).

Large areas sponged at one time allowing for transfer of body heat to the cooling solution. Wet cloths applied to forehead, ankles, wrists, armpits, and groin where blood circulates close to skin surface. Identify temperature to cease treatment due to potential for continued downward temperature drift. Discontinue systemic cold applications and report and document findings if: shivering occurs (this mechanism will raise body temperature); cyanosis of the lips or nails occurs; or accelerated weak pulse occurs

23

Purposes

Control bleeding by constriction of blood vessels. Reduce inflammation; inhibit swelling; decrease pain; and reduce loss of motion at site of inflammation. Control accumulation of fluid. Reduce cellular activity (e.g., check bacterial growth in local infections). Effective initial treatment after trauma (24-48 hours). This application of cold is then frequently followed by a phase of application of heat.

Ice caps or ice collars

Covered with cotton cloth, flannel, or towel to absorb moisture from condensation. Change as needed. Not left on for longer than 1 hour. Cease treatment and report if client complains of cold or numbness, or if area appears mottled.

Cold compresses

Use sterile technique for open wounds. Check site of application after 5-10 minutes for signs of intolerance (cyanosis, blanching, mottling, maceration, or blisters). Remove after prescribed treatment period (usually 20 minutes).

Special considerations

Elderly clients and clients with impaired circulation have decreased tolerance to cold. Moist application of cold penetrates better than dry application.

Application of External Heat

- Rationale
- Relaxes muscles in spasm.
- Softens exudates for easy removal.
- Hastens healing due to vasodilation.
- Localization of infection. (Note: Do not apply heat to the abdomen with
- suspected appendicitis as it may precipitate rupture.)
- Hastens suppuration.
- Warms a body part.
- Reduces congestion of an underlying organ.
- Increases peristalsis.
- Reduces pressure from accumulated fluids.
- Comforts and relaxes.

Dry heat

Hot water bottle/bag, electric heating pad, lamp, cradle, or aquamatic pad. Deeper tissue penetration modes--ultrasound, and shortwave and microwave diathermy (administered by Licensed Physical Therapist).

Follow agency policy for heat application mode ordered: check temperature of water and machine setting carefully; assess site of application frequently for signs of tissue damage or burns; and be alert to potential bleeding resulting from vasodilation.

Moist heat

Soaks, compresses, hot packs. Follow agency policy. Check temperature of application. Use sterile technique for open wounds. Assess skin condition after 5 minutes for increased swelling, excessive redness, blistering, maceration, pronounced pallor, or if the client reports pain or discomfort. Remove the device after 15-25 minutes or as ordered/necessary.

Special considerations

Moist heat penetrates deeper than dry and is usually better tolerated. The skin area involved may vary in any individual depending on the number of heat receptors present. Heat is less tolerated in the very young, elderly, and clients with circulatory problems.

Asepsis

Defined as the absence of disease-producing organisms. Medical asepsis Practices to reduce the number of microorganisms after they leave the body or to reduce transmission.

Often referred to as clean technique.

Includes:

- Hand washing
- Universal or standard precautions
- Isolation technique (see Unit 4)
- Cleaning/disinfecting of equipment.

Surgical asepsis

Practices aimed at destroying pathological organisms before they enter the body through an open wound. Referred to as sterile technique.

Includes: Physical barriers--gloves, masks, gowns, drapes.

High risk procedures:

- Catheter insertion
- Surgical wound dressing changes
- Administration of injections.
- Associated with populations with high risk for infection.

The clients in this category are:

- Transplant recipients
- Burns
- Neonates
- Immunosuppressed/AIDS, cancer clients receiving chemotherapy.

Principles of surgical asepsis

- Sterile field--area where sterile materials for a sterile procedure are placed (e.g., a table covered with sterile drape).
- Sterile field remains sterile throughout procedure.
- Movement in and around field must not contaminate it.
- Keep hands in front of you and above your waist (never reach across the field with unsterile items).
- Barrier techniques (gown, gloves, masks, and drapes are used as indicated to decrease transmission).
- Edges of sterile containers are not sterile once opened.
- Dry field is necessary to maintain sterility of field.

Pressure Sore (Bedsore, Dermal Ulcer, Decubitis Ulcer)

Any lesion caused by unrelieved pressure that causes local interference with circulation and subsequent tissue damage.

Risk factors

- Immobility (e.g.,those with impaired ability to reposition themselves)
- Incontinence
- Impaired nutritional status/intake
- Impaired level of consciousness
- Impaired physical condition (e.g., stability, chronicity, and severity)
- Skin condition impaired (e.g., nourishment, turgor, integrity)
- Predisposing conditions (e.g. diabetes mellitus, neuropathy, vascular disease, anemia, cortisone therapy, etc.)

General prevention, care, and treatment

- Inspect skin and document status and interventions daily.
- Cleanse when soiling occurs (e.g., avoid hot water, harsh, or drying cleansing agents).
- Minimize dry skin (e.g., avoid cold or dry air and use moisturizers as needed).
- Minimize moisture from irritating substances (urine, feces, perspiration,wound drainage).
- Cleanse immediately and apply protective barrier as indicated.
- Avoid massage over bony prominences. (Massage around but not directly over pressure sites.)
- Change position frequently, every 15 minutes to two hours, to decrease prolonged pressure.
- Reduce friction and shearing (e.g., promote lifting rater than dragging).
- Pressure reducing mattresses/beds (e.g., foam, air, gel, or water)
- Positioning devices
- Nutritional intake (especially calories, protein and fluids if not contraindicated).
- Also vitamin A and C, iron and zinc
- ROM, ambulation, or activities as appropriate to promote increased circulation
- Avoid pressure from appliances and care equipment.

Staging of pressure ulcers

Stage I

Observable pressure-related alteration of intact skin as compared to adjacent or opposite area on body. May include changes in color (red, blue, purple tones), temperature (warmth or coolness), skin stiffness (hardness, edema) and/or sensation (pain) (Temporary blanching from pressure can last up to 30 minutes.)

Stage II

Partial thickness loss of skin involving epidermis and/or dermis. Superficial breakdown characterized by blister, abrasion, or shallow crater. Wound base is pink and moist, painful, and free from necrosis.

Stage III

Full thickness skin loss involving subcutaneous damage or necrosis. May extend to but not through underlying fascia. Infection is generally present. Characterized by deep crater or eschar. May include undermining and exudate. Wound base is not usually painful.

Stage IV

Full thickness loss of skin with severe destruction, tissue necrosis, or damage to muscle, bone, or supporting structures (e.g., tendon or joint capsule). Infection, undermining, and sinus tracts are frequently present. If wound contains necrotic tissue or eschar, accurate staging cannot be confirmed until wound base is visible.

Specific wound care treatments

Goals

- Support moist wound healing.
- Prevent or treat infection.
- Avoid trauma of tissue and surrounding skin.
- Comfort
- Solutions
- Cleansing products
- Control of bacteria
- Dressings or coverings

Damp to dry dressing (e.g., gauze dressing put on damp and removed at tacky dry status) debrides slough and scar. If dries completely and adheres to viable tissue, moisten dressing before removal. Non-adherent dressing impregnated with sodium chloride to draw in wound exudate and decrease bacteria. Change at least daily.

Transparent films, semipermeable membrane to promote moist healing by gas exchange and prevention of bacterial and fluid penetration. Change when seal is lost or excessive amount of fluid collected underneath. Hydrocolloid wafers contain water-loving colloids. Wound exudates mixes with wafer to form a gel, moist environment and nonsurgical debridement. Wafers are occlusive and should not be used on infected wounds. Gels/Hydrogels available in sheets or gels and are non adherent. They provide a moist environment and some absorption of bacteria and exudate from the wound.

Not highly absorptive

Do not use on wounds with copious exudate. Be alert to maceration of peri wound areas. (Use moisture barriers.) Exudate absorptive dressings, beads, pastes, or powders which when mixed conform to the wound shape. Attracts debris, exudate, and bacteria via osmosis. Removed only by irrigation. Do not use with deeply undermined wounds or tracts. Foams create a moist environment and absorption.

Nonadherent to wound.

Many require a secondary dressing to secure. Calcium alginates pads or ropes made from seaweed that convert to a firm substance when mixed with exudate.
Highly absorptive--will dry out wounds that have little exudate.

Moisture barrier (e.g., A & D ointment) protects high risk skin from moisture and breakdown. Skin sealant protects high risk skin from moisture and/or chemical breakdown. Debridement--Removal of necrotic devitalized tissue (eschar or slough).

Necrotic tissue provides nutrients for bacterial growth and needs to be removed for healing to occur.

Methods of debridement

Enzymatic
Mechanical
Surgical
Physiologic/autolytic

Be alert to bleeding and damage to adjacent viable tissue.

Miscellaneous

Whirlpool--for cleansing.

Hyperbaric O2-application of high O concentration for healing.
Electrical stimulation--stimulates healing.
Growth factor--cell growth stimulation.

Documentation

Interventions and response to interventions

Address: Location of lesions.

Dimensions--measure and record size (length, width, and depth in cm).

Measuring guides with concentric circles available.

Use sterile applicator to determine accurate depth.

Photographs--need client's written permission.

Stage

Undermining, pockets, or tracts (e.g., undermining from 7:00 to 10:00 measuring 3 cm).

Condition of tissue
- Granulation--red, moist, beefy.
- Epithelialized--new pink, shiny epidermis.
- Necrotic tissue--avascular.
- Slough--yellow, green, gray, brown.
- Eschar--hard, black, leathery.

Drainage

Volume (scant, small, moderate, copious, number of soaked dressings)
Color
Consistency
Odor
Periwound condition and wound margins (e.g., errythema, crepitus, induration, maceration, hematoma, desiccation, blistering, denudation, pustule, tenderness, temperature).
Pain--related to procedures or constant, location, severity.

Nursing Abbreviation Glossary

Letter A Abbreviations ~

- ABG arterial blood gases
- ACE angiotensin converting enzyme
- ACL anterior cruciate ligament
- ACTH adrenocorticotropic hormone
- ADA American Diabetes Association
- ADH antidiuretic hormone
- ADL activities of daily living
- AFB acid-fast bacilli
- AFP alpha-fetoprotein
- AGA appropriate for gestational age
- AIDS acquired immune deficiency syndrome
- AKA above knee amputation
- ALP alkaline phosphatase
- ALT alanine transaminase, alanine aminotransferase
- AMA against medical advice
- AMI acute myocardial infarction
- AODM adult onset diabetes mellitus
- AP apical pulse
- APSGN acute poststreptococcal glomerulonephritis
- ARF acute renal failure
- ASD atrial septal defect
- AST aspartate aminotransferase
- ATN acute tubular necrosis
- AU both ears
- AVB atrio-ventricular block
- A.A. Associate of Arts
- A.A.S. Associate in Applied Science
- A.D. Associate Degree
- A.D.N. Associate Degree in Nursing
- A.S. Associate of Science

Letter B Abbreviations

- BBS bilateral breath sounds
- BE barium enema
- BG blood glucose
- BI brain injury
- BID twice a day
- BILAT bilateral
- B/K below knee
- BM bowel movement or breast milk
- BP blood pressure
- BPH benign prostatic hypertrophy
- BRM biologic response modifiers
- BRP bathroom privileges
- BS bowel sounds
- BSA body surface area
- BSE breast self examination
- BT bowel tones
- BUN blood urea nitrogen
- B.A. Bachelor of Arts
- B.S. Bachelor of Science
- B.S.N. Bachelor of Science in Nursing

Letter C Abbreviations

- C&S culture and sensitivity
- CA calcium, cancer, carcinoma
- CABG coronary artery bypass graft
- CAD coronary artery disease
- CAPD continuous ambulatory peritoneal dialysis
- CAT computerized tomography scan
- CBC complete blood count
- CBD common bile duct
- CBE clinical breast examination
- CBG capillary blood glucose
- CBI continuous bladder irrigation

Letter C Abbreviations

- CBS capillary blood sugar
- CC chief complaint
- CCK cholecystokinin
- CCPD continuous cyclic peritoneal dialysis
- CEA cultured epithelial autograft
- CFT complement-fixation test
- CIN cervical intraepithelial neoplasm
- CL cleft lip
- CMS circulation, motion, sensation
- CO cardiac output
- COPD chronic obstructive pulmonary disease
- CP chest pain, cleft palate
- CPAP continuous positive airway pressure
- CPD cephalo-pelvic disproportion
- CPP cerebral perfusion pressure
- CPPD chest percussion and post drainage
- CRF chronic renal failure
- CRRT continuous renal replacement therapy
- CRT capillary refill time
- CSF cerebrospinal fluid, colony stimulating factors
- CT chest tube, computed tomography
- CVA cerebral vascular accident, costovertebral angle
- CVP central venous pressure
- CX cancel, cervix
- CXR chest x-ray
- CDA Certified Dental Assistant
- CLS Clinical Laboratory Scientist
- CLT Clinical Laboratory Technician
- CMA Certified Medical Assistant
- CNMT Certified Nuclear Medical Technologist
- COTA Certified Occupational Therapy Assistant
- CRTT Certified Respiratory Therapy Technician

Letter D Abbreviations

- DAT diet as tolerated
- DC (dc) discontinue
- DCCT Diabetes Control and Complication Trials
- DEX (DXT) blood sugar
- DIC disseminated intravascular coagulation
- DKA diabetic ketoacidosis
- DNA deoxyribonucleic acid
- DNR do not resuscitate
- DTR deep tendon reflex
- DVT deep vein thrombosis

Letter E Abbreviations

- EBV Epstein-Barr Virus
- ECF extracellular fluid, extended care facility
- EENT eye, ear, nose and throat
- EMC ensephalomyocarditis
- EMG electromyogram
- ERCP endoscopic retrograde cholangiopancreatography
- ESRD end stage renal disease
- ET endotracheal tube
- EMT-B Emergency Medical Technician-Basic
- EMT-I Emergency Medical Technician-Intermediate
- EMT-P Emergency Medical Technician-Paramedic

Letter F Abbreviations

- F & R force and rhythm
- FA fatty acid
- FBS fasting blood sugar
- FD fatal dose, focal distance
- FDA Food & Drug Administration
- FX fracture
- FUO fever of unknown origin
- FVD fluid volume deficit
- FNP Family Nurse Practitioner

Letter G Abbreviations

- GB gallbladder
- GERD gastroesophageal reflux disease
- GFR glomerular filtration rate
- GGT gamma-glutamyl transferase
- GI gastrointestinal
- GOT glutamic oxalic transaminase
- GU genitourinary
- GVHD graft-versus-host-disease

Letter H Abbreviations

- HA headache
- HB hemoglobin
- HCG human chorionic gonadotropin
- HCO3 bicarbonate
- HCT hematocrit
- HD hemodialysis
- HDL high density lipoprotein
- HEENT head, eye, ear, nose and throat
- HGB hemoglobin
- HIV human immunodeficiency virus
- HRT hormone replacement therapy
- HS bedtime
- HX history

Letter I Abbreviations

- IBC iron binding capacity
- IBD inflammatory bowel disease
- IBS irritable bowel syndrome
- IBW ideal body weight
- ICCE intracapsular cataract extraction
- ICF imtermediate care facility
- ICP intracranial pressure
- ICS intercostal space
- ICT inflammation of connective tissue

Letter I Abbreviations

- ICU intensive care unit
- IDM infant of diabetic mother
- IDDM insulin dependent diabetes mellitus
- IE inspiratory exerciser
- IH infectious hepatitis
- IHD ischemic heart disease
- IIP implantable insulin pump
- IM intramuscular
- IMV intermittent mandatory ventilation
- INR international normalization ratio
- IPD intermittent peritoneal dialysis
- IPPB intermittent positive pressure breathing
- ITP immune thrombocytopenic purpura
- IV intravenous
- IVF in vitro fertilization
- IVP intravenous pyelography

Letter J Abbreviations

- JAMA Journal of the American Medical Association
- JVP jugular venous pressure

Letter K Abbreviations

- K potassium
- KCl potassium chloride
- KI potassium iodide
- KUB kidney, ureter, bladder
- KVO keep vein open

Letter L Abbreviations

- L & A light and accommodation
- LAD left anterior descending artery
- LB large bowel
- LDL low density lipoprotein
- LE lupus erythematosus
- LFTs liver function tests
- LIJ left internal jugular
- LLQ left lower quadrant
- LMP last menstrual period
- LP lumbar puncture
- LSC left subclavian
- LUQ left upper quadrant
- LPN Licensed Practical Nurse

Letter M Abbreviations

- MAP mean arterial pressure
- MAR medication administration record
- MCL modified chest lead
- MDI multiple daily vitamin
- MI myocardial infarction
- MLC midline catheter
- MM mucous membrane
- MOABS monoclonal antibodies
- MOM Milk of Magnesia
- MRDD mental retarded/developmentally disabled
- MRI magnetic resonance imaging
- MRM modified radical mastectomy
- MS multiple sclerosis, morphine sulfate
- M.B.A. Master of Business Administration
- M.D. Doctor of Medicine
- M.H.E. Master of Health Education
- M.N. Master of Nursing
- M.P.A. Master of Public Administration
- M.P.H. Master of Public Health

Letter M Abbreviations

- M.P.T. Master of Physical Therapy
- M.S. Master of Science
- M.S.N. Master of Science in Nursing
- M.S.W. Master of Social Work
- MD Medical Doctor
- MLT Medical Laboratory Technician
- MT Medical Technologist

Letter N Abbreviations

- NA sodium
- NACL sodium chloride
- NED no evidence of disease
- NICU neonatal intensive care unit
- NIDDM noninsulin dependent diabetes mellitus
- NKA no known allergies
- NKDA non-ketotic diabetic acidosis
- NKMA no known medcation allergies
- NPD nightly peritoneal dialysis
- NPO nothing by mouth
- NSAID nonsteroidal anti-inflammatory drug
- NTD neural tube defect
- NV nausea & vomiting
- NYD not yet diagnosed

Letter O Abbreviations

- OD right eye
- OGTT oral glucose tolerance test
- ORIF open reduction internal fixation
- OS left eye
- OU both eyes
- OTR Occupational Therapist-Registered

Letter P Abbreviations

- PABA para-aminobenzoic acid
- PC after meals
- PCA patient controlled analgesia, posterior communicating artery
- PCN penicillin, primary care nurse
- PCV packed cell volume
- PD peritoneal dialysis
- PDA patent ductus arteriosus, posterior descending artery
- PDD pervasive development disorder
- PDR physician's desk reference
- PEG percutaneous endoscopic gastrostomy
- PEJ percutaneous endoscopic jejunostomy
- PERL pupils equal, react to light
- PERRLA pupils equal, round, react to light, accommodation
- PET positron emission tomography
- PFT pulmonary function test
- PG prostaglandin
- PH past history
- PI present illness
- PICC peripherally inserted central venous catheter
- PID pelvic inflammatory disease
- PMI point of maximal impulse
- PNH paroxysmal nocturnal hemoglobinuria
- PO by mouth
- PRBC packed red blood cells
- PS pyloric stenosis
- PSA prostate specific antigen
- PT prothrombin time
- PTT partial thromboplastin time
- PUD peptic ulcer disease
- PVD peripheral vascular disease
- PX pneumothorax
- Ph.D. Doctor of Philosophy
- Pharm.D. Doctor of Pharmacy
- PT Physical Therapist
- PTA Physical Therapy Assistant

Letter Q Abbreviations

- QD everyday
- QID four times a day
- QNS quantity not sufficient
- QOD every other day
- QS quantity sufficient, quantity required

Letter R Abbreviations

- RA rheumatoid arthritis
- RAD reactive airway disease
- RAI radioactive iodine
- RAIU radioactive iodine uptake
- RCA right coronary artery
- RDW red cell distribution width
- REEDA redness, edema, ecchymosis, drainage, approximation
- RHD rheumatic heart disease, relative hepatic dullness
- RIJ right internal jugular
- RLQ right lower quadrant
- RM respiratory movement
- ROM range of motion
- ROS review of systems
- RSC right subclavian
- RUQ right upper quadrant
- RX prescription, pharmacy
- RD Registered Dietician
- Registration Abbreviations
- RHIA Registered Health Information Administrator
- RHIT Registered Health Information Technician
- RRA Registered Record Administrator
- RRT Registered Respiratory Therapist
- RT Radiologic Technologist
- RTN Registered Technician of Nuclear Medicine

Letter D Abbreviations

- S/S signs & symptoms
- SAB spontaneous abortion
- SAST serum aspartate aminotransferase
- SB spina bifida
- SBO small bowel obstruction
- SGPT serum glutamic-pyruvic
- transaminase
- SLE systemic lupus erythematosus
- SNF skilled nursing facility

Letter T Abbreviations

- T3 triiodothyronine
- T4 thyroxine
- SOB short of breath
- SR sedimentation rate
- SS social services
- STD sexually transmitted disease
- STH somatotropic hormone
- STM short term memory
- SUI stress urinary incontinence
- SVR systemic vascular resistance
- TBSA total body surface area
- TCDB turn, cough, deep breathe
- TED (hose) thrombo-embolism deterrent
- TEP transesophageal puncture
- THR total hip replacement
- TIA transient ischemic attack
- TIBC total iron binding capacity
- TID three times a day
- TIL tumor infiltrating lymphocytes
- TKR total knee replacement
- TNF tumor necrosis factor
- TNM tumor, node, metastases
-

Letter T Abbreviations

- TNTC too numerous to mention
- TP tuberculin precipitation
- TPN total parenteral nutrition
- TTN transient tachypnea of the newborn
- TTP thrombotic thrombocytopenia purpura
- TUPR trans-urethral prostatic resection
- TUR (or TURP) trans-urethral resection of the prostate
- TWB touch weight bear
- TWE tap water enema
- TX treatment, traction

Letter U, V, W, X, Y, Z Abbreviations

- UA urinalysis
- UAO upper airway obstruction
- UBW usual body weight
- UGI upper gastrointestinal
- UPJ ureteropelvic junction
- URI upper respiratory infection
- US ultrasonic
- UTI urinary tract infection
- UVJ ureterovesical junction
- VA visual acuity
- VBAC vaginal birth after caeserean
- VF ventricular fibrillation
- VLDL very low density lipoprotein
- VMA vanillylmandelic acid
- VSD ventricular septal defect
- VT ventricular tachycardia
- VW vessel wall
- W/C wheelchair
- WBC white blood cell
- WD well developed
- WHO World Health Organization
- WN well nourished
- WNL within normal limits
- XR x-ray
- YO years old
- Z zero

U.S. Hospitals 100 Commonly Diagnosed Medical Disorders –

1. Acne

2. Acquired Immunodeficiency Virus (AIDS) and Human Immunodeficiency Virus (HIV)

3. Acute Respiratory Distress Syndrome (ARDS)

4. Alzheimer's Disease

5. Angina Pectoris

6. Anthrax

7. Arnold-Chiari Malformation

8. Arteriovenous Malformations

9. Arthritis of the Knee

10. Arthritis of the Shoulder

11. Asthma

12. Atherosclerosis

13. Attention Deficit Hyperactivity Disorder (ADHD)

14. Attention Deficit Hyperactivity Disorder (ADHD) - Diagnosis and Treatment

15. Autism

16. Avascular Necrosis (Osteonecrosis)

17. Back Pain I (Conditions)

18. Back Pain II (Diagnosis and Treatment)

19. Benign Prostatic Hyperplasia (BPH)

20. Birth Defects and Developmental Disabilities

21. Birthing Complications: Shoulder Dystocia with Brachial Plexus Injury

22. Brain Anatomy

23. Brain Physiology

24. Brain Trauma - Axonal Shear Injury

25. Breast Cancer

26. Bronchopulmonary Dysplasia (BPD)

27. Burns

28. Cancer of the Uterus (Uterine Cancer)

29. Cardiac Conduction System

30. Cardiomyopathy

31. Care Before and During Pregnancy - Prenatal Care

32. Carpal Tunnel Syndrome

33. Cataract

34. Central Cord Syndrome

35. Central Pain Syndrome

36. Cerebral Aneurysm

37. Cerebral Arteriosclerosis

38. Cerebral Hypoxia

39. Cerebral Palsy Overview

40. Cervical Cancer

41. Chancroid

42. Chiropractic and Its Use in Treating Lower Back Pain

43. Chlamydial Infection

44. Chondromalacia of the Knee Joint

45. Chronic Obstructive Pulmonary Disease (COPD)

46. Cirrhosis of the Liver

47. Colon and Rectal Cancer

48. Constipation

49. Coronary Artery Disease

50. Cushing's Syndrome

51. Cytomegalovirus Infections

52. Deep Vein Thrombosis (DVT) - Blood Clots in the Legs

53. Depression

54. Diabetes

55. Digestive System

56. Down Syndrome

57. Drinking During Pregnancy - Fetal Alcohol Syndrome

58. Emphysema

59. Encephalitis and Meningitis

60. Endometriosis

61. Epidural Pain Relief During Labor Does Not Increase Chance of C-Section

62. Erectile Dysfunction

63. Fibromyalgia

64. Frozen Shoulder (Adhesive Capsulitis)

65. Gallbladder Surgery - Cholecystectomy

66. Gallstones

67. Glaucoma

68. Gonorrhea

69. Group A Streptococcal Infections - Impetigo

70. Group A Streptococcal Infections - Scarlet Fever

71. Group A Streptococcal Infections - Severe

72. Group A Streptococcal Infections - Strep Throat

73. Group A Streptococcal Infections - Cellulitis and Erysipelas

74. Heart Arrhythmia - Rhythm Disorders

75. Heart Attack

76. Heart Bypass Surgery and Coronary Angioplasty Procedure

77. Heart Failure

78. Heart Surgery - Coronary Angioplasty Procedure

79. Heartburn, Hiatal Hernia, and Gastroesophageal Reflux Disease (GERD)

80. High Blood Cholesterol

81. High Blood Pressure

82. High Blood Pressure in Pregnancy - Preeclampsia

83. Hip Replacement

84. Hodgkin's Disease

85. Human Papillomavirus and Genital Warts

86. Human T-Cell Lymphotropic Virus

87. Hydrocephalus

88. Increased Risk of Dying from Pregnancy among Hispanic Women in the United States

89. Inflammatory Breast Cancer

90. Influenza (Flu)

91. Knee and Hip Joint Replacement Surgery (Arthroplasty)

92. Knee Injury - Torn Meniscus (Cartilage)

93. Knee Problems

94. LASIK Eye Surgery

95. Ligament Injuries

96. Ligament Sprains and Strains

97. Lyme Disease

98. Macular Degeneration

99. Malignant Mesothelioma

100.   Melanoma I (Overview)

101.   Melanoma II (Diagnosis and Treatment)

102.   Miscarriage and Stillbirth

103.   Mitral Valve Prolapse

104.   Molluscum Contagiosum

105.   Non-Hodgkin's Lymphoma

106.   Non-Small Cell Lung Cancer

107.   Oral Cancer

108.   Oral Contraceptives and Cancer Risk

109.   Osteoarthritis

110.   Osteochondritis Dissecans

111.   Osteoporosis I- Risk Factors, Prevention

112.   Osteoporosis II - Evaluation and Treatment

113.   Paget's Disease

114.   Parkinson's Disease

NCLEX MASTERS 280 Question Answers and Clinical Reasoning

1. The father of a one-day-old son works the evening shift (3 PM to 11 PM) at another hospital. Which of the following plans would be a priority to meet the needs of this father?

1. Encourage the father to call his wife after work.
2. Instruct the father about visiting policy and suggest AM visitation.
3. Adjust visiting hours to meet the new parents' needs.
4. Present a change of visiting hours to the appropriate hospital committee.

Strategy: Answers are implementation. Determine the outcome of each answer. Is it desired?

(1) Inflexible
(2) inflexible
(3) correct–role of nurse is to be a family and client advocate; this provides individualized care not a priority, although it may be an appropriate long-range goal
(4) not a priority, although it may be an appropriate long-range goal

2. The nurse believes a coworker is diverting narcotics. The nurse approaches the nurse manager to report the suspicions. Which of the following statements by the nurse is BEST?

1. "After my coworker has been on duty, the patients often need repeated doses of pain medication. I have seen her/him sleeping on duty three times."
2. "I saw my coworker downtown after work. S/he was acting really strange, like s/he didn't even recognize me."
3. "I think my coworker is stealing narcotics because s/he is always acting euphoric and seems high."
4. "My coworker is hanging around with drug dealers, and I think I saw tracks on her/his arms."

Strategy: All answers are assessment. Determine how each relates to the situation.

(1) correct—report objective information that can be verified; clues to possible substance abuse by staff include memory lapses, frequent absences from the floor, increased number of clients reporting unrelieved pain or insomnia
(2) subjective observation
(3) subjective observation
(4) "hanging around with drug dealers" is subjective

3. A woman with chronic obstructive pulmonary disease (COPD) is admitted with an acute exacerbation. Her vital signs are: BP 162/100, pulse 78, respirations 30 and labored with wheezing. The nurse should question which of the following orders?

1. Theophylline (Somophyllin) 0.7 mg/kg/hr IV.
2. Tetracycline hydrochloride (Sumycin) 250 mg IM qd.
3. Ipratropium bromide (Atrovent) inhaler 2 inhalations qid.
4. Propranolol hydrochloride (Inderal) 40 mg PO bid.

Strategy:You are looking for an incorrect medication. Think about the action of each drug.

(1) drug of choice for acute asthma
(2) broad spectrum antibiotic, not contraindicated
(3) blocks parasympathetic stimulation and decreases mucus; used with asthma
(4) correct—beta-blocker that blocks beta adrenergic impulses to the bronchial tree that cause bronchodilation resulting in increased bronchoconstriction

4. A husband and wife meet at the mental health clinic to make an appointment for family therapy. Suddenly, the wife begins to sob loudly. As the nurse approaches, the husband says, "I guess we just don't get along." Which of the following responses by the nurse is MOST appropriate?

1. "Your wife seems to be upset by the situation."
2. "Perhaps you should both go home now."
3. "Try to think about what precipitated her crying."
4. "The situation is difficult for both of you."

Strategy: Remember therapeutic communication.

(1) nontherapeutic; emphasis is placed on wife, not the situation

(2) nontherapeutic; closes off communication

(3) nontherapeutic; appears to blame the husband for precipitating the wife's behavior, would cause him to react defensively

(4) correct—therapeutic; avoids blaming, focuses on feelings of both husband and wife

5. A client on chemotherapy has a WBC count of 1,200/mm3. Which of the following nursing actions should the nurse take FIRST?

1. Check temperature q4h.
2. Monitor urine output.
3. Assess for bleeding gums.
4. Obtain an order for blood cultures.

Strategy: Determine how each assessment relates to a low white count.

(1) correct—important to monitor for infection which would be evidenced by an elevated temperature in a client with a low WBC

(2) important because of problems of increased uric acid excretion from chemotherapeutic drugs but should not be done first

(3) would be associated with a low platelet count

(4) done if temperature elevated to determine the type of organism involved

6. A woman is in active labor with her first child when her membranes rupture. She voices a concern to the nurse that she is afraid of having a "dry labor." Which of the following responses by the nurse would be MOST appropriate?

1. "The amniotic fluid provides only minimal lubrication for the labor process."
2. "The amniotic sac may impede the progress of labor and is often ruptured artificially."
3. "Labor is only slightly more difficult with early rupture of the amniotic sac."
4. "Because there is limited amniotic fluid, additional fluids will be supplied."

Strategy: "MOST" indicates there may be more than one answer that you like.

(1) amniotic fluid cushions fetus, allows freedom of movement for musculoskeletal development,
facilitates symmetrical growth, maintains constant body temperature, is a source of oral fluids, and collects wastes

(2) correct—sometimes done to assist or induce labor

(3) does not make labor more difficult

(4) no additional fluids will be supplied

7. The nurse is performing an ice massage for a client in chronic pain. The nurse is MOST concerned if which of the following is observed?

1. Redness or inflammation of the tissue.

2. Mottling or graying of the tissue.

3. The client states that she feels a burning and tingling sensation in the area.

4. The client state that she feels a numbness and a cold sensation in the area.

Strategy: "MOST concerned" indicates a complication.

(1) indicates inflammation

(2) correct—site should be observed every 5 minutes for signs of tissue intolerance, including blanching, mottling, or graying

(3) usually indicates ischemia or sensorineural impairment

(4) expected outcome of numbness, which would lead to decreased pain perception

8. The nurse is caring for a client with a complete heart block. The nurse should question which of the following orders?

1. Administer lidocaine (Xylocaine) 50 mg IV push for PVCs in excess of six per minute.

2. Administer atropine sulfate (Atropine) 0.05 mg IV for symptomatic bradycardia.

3. Anticipate scheduling the client for a temporary pacemaker if the pulse continues to decrease.

4. Mix 10 cc of 1:5,000 solution of isoproterenol (Isuprel) in 500 cc D5W for sustained bradycardia below 30.

Strategy: All answers are implementation. Determine the outcome of each answer. Is it desired?

(1) correct—in complete heart block, the AV node blocks all impulses from the SA node so the atria and ventricles beat independently; because lidocaine suppresses ventricular irritability, it may diminish the existing ventricular response; cardiac depressants are contraindicated in the presence of complete heart block
(2) appropriate treatment
(3) appropriate treatment
(4) appropriate treatment

9. The nurse is caring for a client who had a cholecystectomy. Which of the following observations is MOST important for the nurse to report to the next shift?

1. Resting after receiving IM pain medication.
2. No bowel sounds present.
3. IV infusing at 100 cc/h.
4. Breath sounds decreased in both lower lobes.

Strategy: Priority question. Remember Maslow and the ABCs.

(1) psychosocial; not a priority
(2) physical; expected finding after surgery due to decrease in peristalsis from anesthetic agents
(3) physical; not a priority
(4) correct—physical; incision for a cholecystectomy is high on the abdominal wall, which inhibits ventilatory movement; decreased breath sounds might indicate a complication of pneumonia

10. The nurse in the outpatient clinic plans care for a 65-year-old woman with left-sided weakness due to a cerebral vascular accident (CVA). The client has a history of hypertension and osteoporosis. It is MOST important for the nurse to encourage the client to
1. increase the amount of calcium in her daily diet.
2. increase the amount of vitamin D in her daily diet.
3. increase the amount of time she is exposed to sunlight.
4. increase her activities that involve weight-bearing.

Strategy: All answers are implementation. Determine the outcome of each answer. Is it desired?

(1) diet should have adequate calcium, should increase intake in middle age to protect against skeletal demineralization; not most important

(2) adequate serum levels of vitamin D needed for calcium to be absorbed from GI tract, should increase intake in middle age to protect against skeletal demineralization; not most important

(3) vitamin D is synthesized in the skin with exposure to sunshine; not most important for this patient

(4) correct—weight bearing and exercise primary ways to develop high-density bones, decrease bone reabsorption and stimulate bone formation; would also help maintain mobility with leftsided weakness

11. The homecare nurse is visiting a young adult with a diagnosis of hepatitis A. Which of the following statements, if made by the client to the nurse, indicates that further teaching is needed?

1. "I have been very careful to wash my hands after I go to the bathroom."
2. "I have had to take Tylenol several times this week for this sinus infection I have."
3. "I have been very careful not to handle my child's toys or eating utensils."
4. "My husband has been preparing all of the meals since I've been sick."

Strategy: "Further teaching is needed" indicates you are looking for an incorrect response.

(1) because hepatitis A is spread by the oral-rectal route, it is important to protect others by practicing good hand-washing techniques and avoiding contact with items that will be placed in others' mouths

(2) correct—client should be cautioned about taking any drugs not approved by the health care provider; may become dangerous because of the liver's inability to detoxify and excrete them

(3) because hepatitis A is spread by the oral-rectal route, it is important to protect others by practicing good hand-washing techniques and avoiding contact with items that will be placed in others' mouths

(4) because hepatitis A is spread by the oral-rectal route, it is important to protect others by practicing good hand-washing techniques and avoiding contact with items that will be placed in others' mouths

12. The nurse is caring for a client in a manic phase of bipolar affective disorder. It is MOST important for the nurse to offer which of the following meals?

1. Tuna salad sandwich and orange slices.

2. Bologna sandwich and french fries

3. Milkshake and banana.

4. Fried chicken and tossed salad.

Strategy: All answers are implementations. Determine the outcome of each answer. Is it desired

(1) correct—manic clients need nutritious finger foods; foods contain protein, carbohydrates, vitamin C, and fiber

(2) finger foods, but little nutritive value

(3) finger foods, not as balanced

(4) too difficult to eat in manic phase

13. Which of the following actions should the nurse instruct the client to complete FIRST to establish a normal urinary pattern?

1. Urinate every two hours.

2. Record each time you urinate.

3. Keep a record of your daily fluid intake.

4. Stay near a bathroom.

Strategy: Answers are all implementations. Determine the outcome of each answer. Is it desired?

(1) client should start voiding every 2 h and gradually progress to 3–4 h

(2) second thing to do

(3) correct—client needs to know how much and when he ingests fluid

(4) appropriate, but not the first thing to do.

14. The nurse is receiving reports about four pregnant women in active labor who have been admitted to the labor and delivery unit. Which of the following women should the nurse see FIRST?

1. A 27-year-old nullipara at 38-weeks gestation, has a cervical dilatation of 2 cm, fetus in transverse lie with baseline FHT of 155 bpm.

2. A 32-year-old multipara at term, cervical dilatation of 8 cm, fetus in a vertex presentation with the presenting part at +2 station.

3. A 22-year-old nullipara at term, cervical dilatation of 10 cm, 100% effaced, fetus presenting as left occiput posterior with short-term variability of the FHT at 3–5 beats.

4. A 34-year-old multipara at 37-weeks gestation, has intact amniotic membranes, cervical dilatation of 3 cm, and fetus in a frank breech presentation with the presenting part at station.

Strategy: Determine who is the least stable client.

(1) delivery is not imminent

(2) correct—transition phase of labor and delivery quick for many multipara woman

(3) nullipara women usually have a longer second stage than multipara women

(4) labor has not progressed very far

15. The nurse is planning care for a client who had surgery for an ileal conduit two days ago. It is MOST important for the nurse to take which of the following actions?

1. Remove the appliance regularly and clean the skin with antiseptic solution.

2. Apply a close-fitting drainage bag to the stoma.

3. Massage the skin around the stoma with an emollient.

4. Expose the area around the stoma to air twice a day.

Strategy: Answers are implementations. Determine the outcome of each answer. Is it desired?

(1) soap and water should be used to clean the skin, not an antiseptic solution

(2) correct—primary preventative measure to prevent urine contacting the skin

(3) would hinder the application of the bag for urine collection

(4) unnecessary; would not help prevent skin breakdown

16. Which nursing action is MOST appropriate after intubating a postoperative client who had a respiratory arrest?

1. Soak the intubation equipment in concentrated Betadine solution.
2. Place the intubation blade in a bag and arrange for gas sterilization.
3. Soak the intubation blade in Cidex solution.
4. Wash the equipment with soap and water and allow to air-dry.

Strategy: All answers are implementations. Determine the outcome of each answer. Is it desired?

(1) inappropriate action
(2) correct—equipment sterilization after exposure to body fluids is protocol
(3) inappropriate action
(4) inappropriate action

17. The nurse is caring for a toddler in traction, and the toddler is receiving chloral hydrate (Noctec). The toddler becomes irritable and extremely restless. Which nursing action is MOST appropriate?

1. Give the next dose of chloral hydrate early.
2. Contact the physician to obtain new orders.
3. Instruct the toddler's mother to read to him.
4. Take the toddler out of traction for 30 minutes.

Strategy: All answers are implementations. Determine the outcome of each answer. Is it desired?

(1) would probably increase the restlessness and worsen the condition by giving the toddlermore medication
(2) correct—chloral hydrate, a sedative, can have the opposite effect on a toddler, causing excitability
(3) restless due to chloral hydrate
(4) toddler should remain in traction

18. The nurse performs diet teaching for a client with a spinal cord injury at S-3. Which of the following meals, if chosen by the client, would indicate to the nurse that teaching has been effective?

1. Cheeseburger with tomato and onion.
2. Spaghetti with meat sauce and green beans.
3. Tuna fish sandwich with orange juice.
4. Grilled cheese sandwich and chocolate pudding.

Strategy: Type of diet needed by the client is unstated. Determine what type of diet is required and select the appropriate menu.
(1) should have high-fiber, low-fat diet; this diet is high in fat
(2) correct—high-fiber diet is an important part of bowel program; fiber helps prevent the complication of constipation; includes whole-grain foods, bran, fresh and dried fruits; increased fiber will facilitate defecation, with reduction in fat intake
(3) should increase intake of fiber foods and decrease intake of fat
(4) should have high-fiber, low-fat diet; this is a high-fat diet

19. The nurse is screening an eight-month-old girl in a well-baby clinic. The nurse would be MOST concerned if the infant's mother made which of the following statements?

1. "My daughter has almost doubled her birth weight."
2. "When I walk in the room my child smiles at me."
3. "When she is around her grandpa, my child cries."
4. "My daughter can't quite say Mama yet."

Strategy: "MOST concerned" indicates you are looking for something wrong.
(1) correct—weight should double by 5 months
(2) begins to recognize parents at 6 months
(3) begins to fear strangers at 6 months, increases until 9 months
(4) begins to say "dada" and "mama" with meaning at 10 months

20. A 16-year-old young woman is brought by her parents to the outpatient clinic for treatment of pelvic inflammatory disease (PID). While the nurse obtains a history, the client says bitterly, "My parents are mean and don't really care about me." Which of the following responses by the nurse is BEST?

1. "You feel your parents don't care about you?"
2. "Your parents brought you to the clinic, didn't they?"
3. "I am sure that your parents have your best interests at heart."
4. "Did you have a disagreement with your parents?"

Strategy: Remember the principles of therapeutic communication.
(1) correct—uses therapeutic technique of reflecting; validates feelings without placing value judgment or giving approval or disapproval
(2) negates client's feelings, blocks communication
(3) negates client's feelings, blocks communication
(4) yes/no question

21. A 55-year-old woman with end-stage metastatic cancer of the breast is admitted to the hospital. It is MOST important for the nurse to
1. suction the patient frequently.
2. provide an air mattress.
3. turn the patient every two hours.
4. give the patient frequent baths.

Strategy: All answers are implementations. Determine the outcome of each answer. Is it desired?
(1) decreases oxygen levels, is uncomfortable and unnecessary
(2) equipment is not most important
(3) correct—prevents complications such as skin breakdown
(4) will dry out her skin and cause chilling

22. One hour after receiving 7 U of regular insulin, the client presents with diaphoresis, pallor, and tachycardia. The priority nursing action would be to
1. notify the physician.
2. call the lab for a blood glucose level.
3. offer the client milk and crackers.
4. administer glucagon.

Strategy: Answers are a mix of assessments and implementations. Does this situation require validation? No. Determine the outcome of each implementation.

(1)action should be taken prior to notifying the physician

(2) does not require validation, implementation required

(3) correct—onset of action for regular insulin is 30–60 minutes; assessment indicates a problem with hypoglycemia; foods such as milk and crackers should be given if blood sugar is around 40–60 mg/dL; if orange juice or simple sugar is given, it should be followed with a meal or with protein intake

(4) unnecessary, unless client is unresponsive

23. An 11-month-old baby is having trouble gaining weight after discharge from the hospital. Which of the following actions by the nurse is BEST?

1. Observe the child at mealtime.
2. Inquire about the child's eating patterns.
3. Weigh the baby each month.
4. Attempt to feed the baby for the mother.

Strategy: Answers are a mix of assessments and implementations. Is validation required? Yes.

(1) correct—assessment; will provide the most information

(2) assessment; may or may not secure an accurate picture

(3) assessment; weight should be obtained more often or on each visit

(4) implementation; need to assess before determining appropriate interventions

24. A client has been receiving chlorpromazine (Thorazine) 400 mg/day for four weeks. He experiences an oral temperature of 105°F (40.5°C), severe rigidity, oculogyric crisis, and severe hypertension. It is MOST important for the nurse to take which of the following actions?

1. Administer PRN benztropine mesylate (Cogentin) immediately.
2. Hold the chlorpromazine and notify the medical staff stat.
3. Place the client in isolation on bedrest in semi-Fowler's position.
4. Administer acetaminophen 500 mg and place the client on a cooling mattress.

Strategy: All answers are implementations. Determine the outcome of each answer. Is it desired?

(1) bromocriptine (Parlodel) or dantrolene (Dantrium) is used for CNS toxicity

(2) correct—client is experiencing neuroleptic malignant syndrome; fatal in about 15–20% of cases; is toxic effect of antipsychotic medication

(3) isolation is unnecessary

(4) is not most important; cooling blanket is used for fever, IV fluids for hydration, airway if necessary, frequent monitoring of vital signs

25. A 32-year-old man comes to the clinic for a glycosylated hemoglobin assay (HbA1c). The result is 6%. The nurse should

1. document the findings in the chart.
2. call the physician about orders to adjust the insulin dosage.
3. give him 15 g of carbohydrates.
4. ask him to list the foods he has eaten in the last 24 hours.

Strategy: Answers are a mix of assessments and implementations. Does this situation require validation? No. Determine the outcome of each answer choice.

(1) correct—results normal, indicates good control of diabetes

(2) no adjustments need to be made

(3) does not reflect hypoglycemia

(4) no adjustment needs to be made in diet; result is not altered by intake day before test

26. A school-aged child informs the school nurse that his right knee "doesn't feel right." Which of the following actions should the nurse take FIRST?

1. Instruct the child to extend the right leg.
2. Put both of the child's legs through range-of-motion.
3. Advise the child to soak the right knee in warm water.
4. Compare the appearance of the right knee with the left knee.

Strategy: Answers are a mix of assessments and implementations. Does this situation require assessment? Yes. Is there an appropriate assessment? Yes.

(1) will not help determine if the knee is edematous

(2) inspection first step of physical assessment

(3) implementation; need to assess to determine the problem

(4) correct—should compare corresponding joints for symmetry and to determine normal

parameters

27. The nurse is caring for a client receiving treatment for hypoparathyroidism. The nurse determines that treatment has been successful if which of the following was observed?

1. The client's output is 1500 cc of clear straw-colored urine.

2. The client is unable to state his name.

3. The client denies numbness and tingling.

4. The client loses 3 pounds in one week

Strategy: Determine how each answer relates to hypoparathyroidism.

(1) important to monitor, but are not top priority

(2) confusion and decreased memory are symptoms of hypercalcemia

(3) correct—tetany is major sign of hypoparathyroidism

(4) most frequently observed with hyperparathyroidism

28. The nurse in the newborn nursery receives report from the previous shift. Which of the following infants should the nurse see FIRST?

1. A two-day-old infant, lying quietly alert, heart rate of 185 bpm.

2. A one-day-old infant, crying, and the anterior fontanel is bulging.

3. A 12-hour-old infant, held by the mother, respirations 45 and irregular.

4. A five-hour-old infant, sleeping, hands and feet are blue bilaterally.

Strategy: Eliminate the stable patients.

(1) correct—infant has tachycardia; normal resting rate is 120–160; requires further investigation

(2) crying causes increased intracranial pressure, causes fontanel to bulge

(3) normal respiratory rate is 30–50 breaths per minute with apneic episodes

(4) acrocyanosis is normal for 2–6 hours post delivery due to poor peripheral circulation

29. The nurse plans care for a 36-year-old woman with Graves' disease. The nurse knows that which of the following foods or fluids should be restricted for this client?

1. Milk.

2. Apples.

3. Orange juice.

4. Tea.

Strategy: Think about each answer.

(1) not limited for Graves' disease

(2) not limited for Graves' disease

(3) not limited for Graves' disease

(4) correct—stimulant that would increase metabolic rate

30. After the anesthesiologist administers an epidural to a woman in labor, which of the following nursing actions has the HIGHEST priority?

1. Decrease IV fluids.

2. Assess the fetal heart monitor.

3. Place the mother on her right side.

4. Obtain the blood pressure.

Strategy: Answers are a mix of assessments and implementations. Does this situation require assessment? Yes. Is there an appropriate assessment? Yes.

(1) implementation; client must be well hydrated before and after the procedure

(2) assessment; may be done as ongoing management, but is not a priority

(3) implementation; laboring mother placed on left side to promote uterine perfusion

(4) *correct*—assessment; side effect of an epidural is hypotension from the vasodilation that occurs

31. A client is being followed in the rape-crisis clinic one week after being assaulted. The client is currently taking Xanax 0.25 mg PO q6h for anxiety. Which of the following statements, if made by the client to the nurse, reflects a *correct* understanding of this medication?

1. "I can take it whenever I feel upset."
2. "I should not take this with anything but water."
3. "I guess I need to stop drinking white wine."
4. "This medication will help me forget and go on."

Strategy: All answers are implementations. Determine the outcome of each answer. Is it desired?

(1) indicates a need for further medication teaching

(2) indicates a need for further medication teaching

(3) *correct*—sedative drugs should not be taken with alcoholic beverages

(4) indicates a need for further medication teaching

32. The nurse is caring for clients in a rehabilitation facility. The nursing team reports that a client recovering from a hip fracture has repeatedly "transferred herself to the floor." Which of the following actions, if taken by the nurse, is BEST?

1. Place the call light within the client's reach.
2. Remove the footrests from the wheelchair.
3. Observe the client trying to rise from a sitting to a standing position.
4. Place a posey vest restraint on the client.

Strategy: Answers are a mix of assessments and implementations. Does this situation require assessment? Yes. Is there an appropriate assessment? Yes.

(1) implementation; assumes that client can't reach the call light

(2) implementation; assumes that client is tripping on the footrest

(3) *correct*—assessment; nurse can determine if client is safe to perform this activity.

(4) implementation; must exhaust all other interventions before restraining client

33. A client had a thoracotomy 3 hours ago. For the past 2 hours there has been 100 cc per hour of bloody chest drainage. Which of the following actions should the nurse take FIRST?

1. Increase the IV fluid rate.
2. Administer oxygen at 5 L/min per oxygen mask.
3. Elevate the head of the bed.
4. Advise the physician of the amount of drainage.

Strategy: All answers are implementations. Determine the outcome of each answer. Is it desired?

(1) may be appropriate after the physician is notified
(2) may be appropriate after the physician is notified
(3) may be appropriate after the physician is notified
(4) *correct*—chest drainage of 100 cc/hr is abnormal; physician should be notified

34. While a client is receiving TPN, it is MOST important for the nurse to monitor

1. vital signs and level of consciousness.
2. arterial blood gases and liver enzymes.
3. serum glucose and electrolytes.
4. skin turgor and daily weights.

Strategy: "MOST important" indicates a priority question.

(1) most common complications involve fluid and electrolytes
(2) abnormalities in liver function may occur, but most common complications involve fluid and electrolytes
(3) *correct*—hyperglycemia can cause diuresis and excessive fluid loss; should check fingerstick blood sugar every 6 h, check serum electrolytes (sodium, potassium, calcium, magnesium, phosphates) several times a week
(4) not most important; should assess skin turgor to check for dehydration and weigh daily

35. The physician prescribes sulfisoxazole (Gantrisin) 2 g PO qid for a client. Which of the following instructions is MOST important for the nurse to include when teaching the client about this medication?

1. "Drink plenty of fluids."
2. "Wear sunscreen when outdoors."
3. "Eliminate dairy products from your diet."
4. "Take this medication with meals."

Strategy: All answers are implementations. Determine the outcome of each answer. Is it desired?

(1) *correct*—prevents crystalluria and stone formation
(2) sun sensitivity not seen with this medication
(3) no dietary restrictions with medication
(4) if given with meals, it delays but doesn't interfere with amount of medication absorbed

36. The nurse on postpartum is preparing four clients for discharge. It would be MOST important for the nurse to refer which of the following clients for homecare?

1. A 15-year-old who vaginally delivered a 7-lb male two days ago.
2. An 18-year-old multipara who delivered a 9-lb female by cesarean section two days ago.
3. A 20-year-old multipara who delivered 1 day ago and is complaining of cramping.
4. A 22-year-old who delivered by cesarean section and is complaining of burning on urination.

Strategy: Eliminate the most stable patients.

(1) stable situation, no indication of problems with mother or baby
(2) stable situation, no indication of problems with mother or baby
(3) stable patient, cramping due to uterine contractions
(4) *correct*—unstable patient, indicates urinary tract infections; requires follow-up

37. The client is to receive regional anesthesia (spinal anesthesia) during surgery. Which of the following is an important nursing implication regarding this anesthesia?

1. The client should be adequately hydrated in order to prevent hypotension after anesthesia is established.
2. To decrease the risk of aspiration, the client must be NPO at least 12 hours prior to the initiation of the anesthesia.
3. Assess the client for any allergies to Betadine or iodine preparations.
4. Determine specific gravity of the urine,prepare client for insertion of a central line.

Strategy: Answers are a mix of assessments and implementations. Do the assessments make sense? No.
(1) *correct*—implementation; important that the client be well hydrated to prevent hypotensive
problems after the spinal anesthesia is initiated
(2) implementation; unnecessary for client to be NPO for 12 hours
(3) assessment; unnecessary, as iodine dyes are not used
(4) assessment/implementation; irrelevant to the procedure

38. A client has a cataract removed from the left eye. Which of the following is an important nursing intervention in the immediate postoperative period?

1. Position the client on the right side with the head slightly elevated.
2. Place the client on the left side to protect the eye.
3. Perform sensory neurological checks every two hours.
4. Maintain complete bedrest for the first 48 hours.

Strategy: Answers are all implementations. Determine the outcome of each answer choice. Is it desired?
(1) *correct*—should be positioned on back or unaffected side to prevent trauma to surgical eye
(2) should be positioned on unaffected side
(3) unnecessary for cataract clients
(4) unnecessary for cataract clients

39. A 48-year-old woman is diagnosed with a tumor of the pituitary gland and has a transsphenoidal hypophysectomy. The nurse plans care for the patient two days after surgery. It is MOST important for the nurse to monitor the patient's

1. complete blood count (CBC).
2. temperature.
3. specific gravity of urine.
4. intracranial pressure.

Strategy: "MOST important" indicates that this is a priority question. Determine what each assessment measures and how it relates to the situation.

(1) not affected by surgery

(2) controlled by the medulla, not the pituitary

(3) *correct*—lack of ADH from pituitary will cause diabetes insipidus and diuresis with very low

specific gravity

(4) surgery performed through nose; does not affect cerebral pressure

40. A 68-year-old client has an order for hydrochlorothiazide (Hydrodiuril) 50 mg qd. The nurse knows that teaching has been successful if the client makes which of the following statements?

1. "I should not operate heavy machinery."
2. "I should drink only drink five glasses of liquid per day."
3. "This medication will cause my urine to turn orange."
4. "I should eat dried apricots each day."

Strategy: All answers are implementations. Determine the outcome of each answer. Is it desired?

(1) medication does not cause drowsiness

(2) there are no specific restrictions on fluid at this time

(3) does not occur

(4) *correct*—continued use of this diuretic may cause a loss of potassium; dietary intake of foodssuch as bananas or dried apricots, which are high in potassium, should be encouraged

41. A LPN/LVN contacts the nurse to say that s/he has shingles on her/his back. Which of the following statements by the nurse is BEST?

1. "You can't take care of clients for fourteen days."
2. "Come to work as scheduled."
3. "You can't care for clients until the lesions are crusted."
4. "Please contact your physician."

Strategy: The topic of the question is unstated. Read answer choices for clues.

(1) staff with localized lesions can care for non–high risk clients
(2) *correct*—able to care for non–high risk clients; cover lesions
(3) can't care for immunosuppressed clients until lesions have crusted
(4) passing the buck

42. The infant of a diabetic mother has a blood glucose of 90 mg/dL and a serum calcium level of 7.0 mg/dL. The nurse should anticipate that which of the following medications would be administered IV?

1. Insulin.
2. Glucose.
3. Phenobarbital.
4. Calcium gluconate.

Strategy: Determine the action of each drug and how it relates to the lab values.

(1) would be given for blood sugar problems
(2) would be given for blood sugar problems
(3) not appropriate for a neonate
(4) *correct*—hypocalcemia causes tetany; calcium gluconate will replace the calcium

43. The nurse is performing hypertension screening at the local grocery store. It would be MOST important for the nurse to complete which of the following tasks?

1. Use a blood pressure cuff that overlaps the arm at least four inches.
2. Support the client's arm above the level of the heart.
3. Take two readings at least five minutes apart.
4. Take the blood pressure after the client has exercised for 10 minutes.

Strategy: All answers are implementations. Determine the outcome of each answer choice. Is it desired?

(1) unnecessary

(2) arm should be supported at the level of the heart

(3) *correct*—recognition of adult hypertension should be done after two readings taken at least

five minutes apart

(4) unnecessary

44. Which of the following indicates that a client is beginning to develop a trusting relationship with the nurse?

1. The client describes delusions to the nurse.
2. The client can describe his/her feelings to the nurse.
3. The nurse feels more comfortable with the client.
4. The client reports feeling less anxious.

Strategy: Think about each answer. Does the behavior indicate trust?

(1) delusional system is indication of anxiety, delusions will increase with greater anxiety; trust of nurse is not related to an explanation of client's delusions

(2) *correct*—client who is suspicious and delusional begins to demonstrate trusting behaviors when s/he shares feelings with the nurse

(3) nurse's response can be an indication of transference/counter-transference issues; is not indicative of client beginning to enter a trusting relationship

(4) is beneficial that the client's anxiety level is becoming less intense; will facilitate development of a trusting relationship

45. The nurse is caring for a client with a long leg cast on his right leg. The nurse notes that the right foot is pale and cool to the touch, and the client continues to complain of pain even though an analgesic was administered 45 minutes ago. What is the FIRST action the nurse should take?

1. Apply a heating pad to the client's right toes.
2. Repeat the dose of the analgesic stat.
3. Remove the cast immediately.
4. Notify the physician immediately.

Strategy: All answers are implementations. Determine the outcome of each answer. Is it desired?

(1) inappropriate response to the symptoms observed

(2) it is not likely that the analgesic was ordered q 45 min; is only palliative

(3) is the action that probably will be done by the physician

(4) *correct*—symptoms of compartmental syndrome; document observations and secure physician's intervention immediately

46. The nurse is caring for a client after dental surgery. The dentist has prescribed ibuprofen (Motrin IB) 600 mg PO. The nurse would be MOST concerned if the client made which of the following statements?

1. "I was treated for a peptic ulcer two years ago."
2. "I had a transurethral resection of the prostate (TURP) last year."
3. "I attend Weight Watchers."
4. "I have been having problems with gout."

Strategy: Determine how each statement relates to ibuprofen.

(1) *correct*—side effects include epigastric distress, nausea, occult blood loss, peptic ulceration;
use cautiously with history of previous GI disorders

(2) medication not contraindicated

(3) medication not contraindicated

(4) medication not contraindicated

47. The nurse is obtaining a health history on a client in the medical clinic. The client states, "I think I have an ulcer." Which of the following responses by the nurse is BEST?

1. "Do you have a burning pain in the epigastric region?"
2. "Do you have sharp pain in your lower abdomen?"
3. "Do you have right shoulder pain with vomiting?"
4. "Do you have heartburn when you lie down?"

Strategy: Determine how each answer relates to an ulcer.
(1) *correct*—peptic ulcer pain is often referred to as a "boring pain in the back," or a "burning, gnawing" feeling in the midepigastric area
(2) may indicate intestinal perforation
(3) often associated with gallbladder disease or with irritation of the diaphragm, most often
caused by free air in abdominal cavity (a postoperative complication)
(4) describes indigestion or possible hiatal hernia

48. The nurse is caring for a neonate with an infection. The nurse would be MOST concerned if which of the following was observed?

1. Heart rate of 150 bpm.
2. Axillary temperature of 96°F (35.5°C).
3. Weight increase of 4 oz.
4. Respiratory rate of 65 at rest.

Strategy: Determine how each answer relates to neonatal infection.

(1) is within the normal range
(2) is not significant
(3) neonates normally experience a five to ten percent loss of weight within the first few days of life
(4) *correct*—normal respiratory rate of a neonate is 30–50; tachypnea is a sign of sepsis or hypoxia in a neonate

49. An involuntary psychiatric patient asks the nurse to mail his letter to the President. He states that the letter will make the President regret his actions to prevent homosexuals from serving in the military. Which of the following responses by the nurse is BEST?

1. Accept the letter and place it in the patient's medical record.
2. Read the patient's letter and decide if it is appropriate to mail.
3. Call the patient's psychiatrist and inform him of the letter.
4. Discourage the patient from sending the letter, but mail it if patient insists.

Strategy: All answers are implementations. Determine the outcome of each answer. Is it desired?
(1) psychiatric patients do not forfeit their civil rights
(2) patient has the right to send and receive unopened mail
(3) has the right to mail the letter
(4) *correct*—retains the right to communicate with elected officials

50. During administration of oral medications to an elderly, confused client, the client states, "These pills look funny. They belong to the lady down the hall." Which of the following is the BEST response by the nurse?

1. "Your physician has ordered new medications for you. They will help you get well."
2. "Remember yesterday when I brought your medications? They look the same."
3. "I'll explain why you are receiving these medications."
4. "I'll be back after I check your medications again."

Strategy: All answers are implementations. Determine the outcome of each answer. Is it desired?
(1) unsafe action
(2) unsafe action
(3) unsafe action
(4) *correct*—even confused client should have his/her medications rechecked when there is any possibility of an error; always observe the five rights of medication administration

51. The nurse discusses symptoms of the onset of labor with a 26-year-old primipara. Which of the following statements, if made by the client to the nurse, indicates a need for further teaching?

1. "I will note an increase in fetal movement."
2. "I may feel a gush of fluid run down my legs."
3. "I may see some blood in my vaginal discharge."
4. "I may experience a low backache."

Strategy: " Need for further teaching" indicates you are looking for an in *correct* **response.**

(1) *correct*—usually movement decreases with the onset of labor
(2) indicates rupture of membranes, symptom of labor
(3) bloody show is symptom of labor
(4) symptom of labor

52. At a health-screening clinic, an adult male client's total plasma cholesterol level is 200 mg/dL. Which of the following actions by the nurse is BEST?

1. Refer the client to a doctor for appropriate medication.
2. Refer the client to the dietitian.
3. Obtain a diet history.
4. Recheck the cholesterol level in two years.

Strategy: Answer choices are a mix of assessments and implementations. Does this situation require assessment? Yes.

(1) implementation; levels higher than 250 mg/dL may require medication if diet therapy is not effective
(2) implementation; passing the buck
(3) *correct*—assessment; total cholesterol level for an adult male should be under 200 mg/dL;higher levels require a low-fat diet; obtain diet history before instructing on a low-fat diet
(4) assessment; blood level should be checked earlier than two years

53. In working with an overweight adolescent with hypertension, the most helpful suggestion the nurse should make regarding long-term health promotion and maintenance would be to

1. avoid participating in organized sports.
2. join an adolescent weight reduction support group.
3. limit socialization with friends of normal weight.
4. adhere to a 1,000-calorie low-fat diet.

Strategy: Answers are implementations. Determine the outcome of each answer. Is it desired?

(1) properly supervised physical activity is desirable, not to be avoided
(2) *correct*—excellent means of obtaining information and support for the client
(3) isolation from peers should be avoided
(4) does not supply enough calories for an adolescent

54. A nurse is caring for client immediately after abdominal aortic aneurysm repair. Vitals are: blood pressure 100/70, pulse 120, respirations 24, urine output 75 cc for 3 hours. Which is priority nursing action(s) for this client?

1. Weigh the client.
2. Obtain an EKG.
3. Decrease the rate of the IV fluids and start nasal oxygen.
4. Maintain bedrest and evaluate for a decrease in CVP readings.

Strategy: Determine what the problem is in the stem (shock). Determine how each answer relates to shock.

(1) not a priority
(2) an EKG will not determine cause of tachycardia
(3) rate of IV fluids will most likely be increased
(4) *correct*—client is at increased risk for development of hypovolemic shock; vital signs and urine output correlate with the early signs of shock; the nurse should compare the CVP with previous readings

55. The nurse is performing teaching on a client who is receiving isoniazide (INH) 300 mg PO qd. The nurse identifies that teaching has been successful if the client makes which of the following statements?

1. "My urine will turn brown."
2. "I will take this medication for two weeks."
3. "I shouldn't take any other medication while taking this drug."
4. "I should not drink any alcoholic beverages."

Strategy: Determine how each answer relates to INH.
(1) untrue statement
(2) untrue statement
(3) untrue statement
(4) *correct*—alcohol consumption while on INH therapy has been reported to increase isoniazidrelated hepatitis; clients should be cautioned to restrict consumption of alcohol

56. A 14-year-old client is admitted for insertion of a Harrington rod due to scoliosis. In preparation for the immediate postoperative care, the nurse should include which of the following in a teaching plan for this client?

1. Take ten deep breaths every two hours.
2. Get on the bedpan by lifting the hips.
3. Soft diet as tolerated.
4. Elevate legs ten times every four hours.

Strategy: All answers are implementations. Determine the outcome of each answer. Is it desired?
(1) *correct*—clients must be monitored closely for the first 48 to 72 hours for respiratory
problems; bowel and urinary problems need to be assessed along with neurological problems in the extremities
(2) client will have a catheter
(3) client may have a nasogastric tube connected to low suction
(4) not appropriate for the situation

57. The nurse learns that a staff member providing care to a client with cytomegalovirus is in early pregnancy. Which of the following actions, if taken by the nurse, is BEST?

1. Reassign the pregnant staff member to care for other patients.
2. Instruct the staff member to contact her physician.
3. Ask the staff member how she is feeling about her pregnancy.
4. Ensure that the staff member follows standard precautions.

Strategy: Answers are a mix of assessments and implementations. Is validation required? No. Determine the outcome of each implementation.

(1) no reason to reassign the staff member

(2) passing the buck

(3) discuss nurse's feeling about caring for high-risk clients, but is not the priority

(4) *correct*—make pregnant personnel aware of the risks; use standard precautions, do not reassign

58. The nurse encounters a psychotic client coming out of his room nude. Which of the following responses by the nurse is BEST?

1. "Come with me, Mr. Jones. You need to get dressed."
2. "Why are you coming into the hallway undressed, Mr. Jones?
3. "Being naked in the hallway is inappropriate, Mr. Jones. Return to your room to get dressed."
4. "Do I need to get a male nurse to help you get dressed, Mr. Jones?"

Strategy: Remember therapeutic communication.

(1) inappropriate behavior must be explained to client

(2) don't ask "why" questions

(3) *correct*—identifies inappropriate behavior and tells client what change must take place

(4) yes/no question

59. A patient on suicide precautions asks for a razor to shave her legs. When the nurse tells the patient s/he must remain with the patient, the patient responds, "Don't you trust me?" Which of the following responses by the nurse is BEST?

1. "It is against hospital policy to allow patients on suicide precautions to have razors unsupervised."
2. "I trust you, but your doctor said a nurse has to watch you if you want to shave your legs."
3. "Wouldn't you rather wait until you are feeling better before you try and shave your legs?"
4. "You have been having thoughts about wanting to hurt yourself recently, so I'll stay with you."

Strategy: Remember therapeutic communication.
(1) true statement, but not the most therapeutic
(2) passing the buck
(3) yes/no question
(4) *correct*—provides patient with factual information in a caring manner

60. A 76-year-old woman has a medical history that includes hypertension with cardiac involvement. A public health nurse visits this client regularly and on each visit records her vital signs. Which of the following findings would the nurse expect for this client?

1. Temperature 99.5°F (37.5°C), pulse 110, respirations 32, blood pressure 140/80.
2. Temperature 98.6°F (37°C), pulse 78, respirations 16, blood pressure 120/80.
3. Temperature 99.8°F (37.7°C), pulse 90, respirations 20, blood pressure 150/90.
4. Temperature 96.8°F (36°C), pulse 80, respirations 20, blood pressure 160/90.

Strategy: All answers are assessments. Determine how each relates to the situation. Remember the "comma, comma, and" rule.
(1) temperature, pulse, and respirations too high for the elderly
(2) would expect with younger client without history of hypertension
(3) temperature and pulse elevated; not expected with elderly clients
(4) *correct*—temperature is usually lower due to decrease in BMR, pulse and respirations normal, BP expected with history of hypertension

61. A 74-year-old man is brought by his daughter to the emergency room. When asked his name he is unable to remember it, and appears to be disheveled, restless, and confused. His daughter says she has been caring for him at home for the last year, but he "ran away" after they had an argument about his deteriorating personal hygiene. She found him several hours later sitting in the street. She confides to the nurse that she feels horrible about yelling at her father.

Which of the following is the BEST response by the nurse?
1. "We all do things that we are sorry for later."
2. "Don't feel guilty because he is confused."
3. "Your father's illness must be difficult for both of you."
4. "The social worker will be able to help you with this problem."

Strategy: Remember therapeutic communication.

(1) closed statement; doesn't encourage discussion of feelings

(2) minimizes feelings and problems; nontherapeutic

(3) *correct*—responds to feeling tone, encourages discussion of feelings

(4) passing the buck; doesn't respond to feeling tone

62. The nurse is supervising care of a group of children in a day care facility. The nurse would intervene in which of the following situations?

1. A 4-year-old is given paper to write to a pen pal.
2. A 7-year-old is playing with an electric train set.
3. A 9-year-old is performing magic tricks for his friends.
4. A 12-year-old discusses collecting canned goods for the holidays.

Strategy: Remember growth and development milestones.

(1) *correct*—task too advanced for a preschooler

(2) appropriate for this age group

(3) helps cognitive development of child

(4) appropriate for this age group

63. A dying client is on a unit with limited visiting hours that restrict children under 12 years from visiting. Which nursing action has the HIGHEST priority

1. Explain the visiting hours to the client's family.
2. Propose a policy change to the medical and nursing staff.
3. Allow flexibility with family members' visitation.
4. Encourage the family to call the unit between visiting hours.

Strategy: Answers are implementations. Determine the outcome of each answer. Is it desired?
(1) does not address the client's needs
(2) not highest priority
(3) *correct*—role of the nurse is to function as client advocate; is important to individualize care with all clients
(4) does not address the client's needs

64. A client is diagnosed with otosclerosis and is admitted for a stapedectomy. It is MOST important for the nurse to ask which of the following questions?

1. "Have you noticed fluid draining from your left ear?"
2. "Have you had problems hearing for your entire life?"
3. "Did you require speech therapy when you were a child?"
4. "When did you notice that your hearing was impaired?"

Strategy: Determine how each answer relates to otosclerosis.
(1) describes ruptured tympanic membrane, not relevant to otosclerosis
(2) hearing impairment may begin in the early adult years, but not at birth
(3) speech is not affected by hearing loss
(4) *correct*—otosclerosis occurs gradually over many years; often client is not aware of it until the impairment is significant

65. The nurse is obtaining a health history from a client taking phenytoin sodium (Dilantin). It would be MOST important for the nurse to report which of the following client statements to the physician?

1. "I've had several 'blackouts' in the past year."
2. "My mother has seizures, but this medication does not work for her."
3. "I don't know when I had my last menstrual period."
4. "I took this medicine several years ago but stopped when my urine turned pink."

Strategy: Determine the significance of each answer and how it relates to Dilantin.

(1) not relevant to this medication

(2) not relevant to this medication

(3) *correct*—phenytoin sodium (Dilantin) is in pregnancy risk category D; doctor should be

notified of the possibility of a pregnancy

(4) pink urine is a normal occurrence when taking Dilantin

66. A client is being treated for thrombophlebitis with heparin sodium infusion at 800 U/h. The nurse would be MOST concerned if which of the following was observed?

1. Increased anxiety.
2. Decreased heart rate.
3. Increased partial thromboplastin time.
4. Decreased level of consciousness.

Strategy: "MOST concerned" indicates a complication.

(1) in *correct*

(2) in *correct*

(3) desired response to therapy

(4) *correct*—major side effect is intracranial bleeding; decrease in level of consciousness is first sign

67. The nurse is caring for a client with a CVA with right-sided paralysis. It would be MOST appropriate for the nurse to take which of the following actions?

1. Insert a Foley catheter.
2. Assist the client to ambulate three times per day.
3. Determine if assistance is needed with feeding.
4. Position the client on the right side.

Strategy: Answers are a mix of assessments and implementations. Is the assessment appropriate? Yes.

(1) not required unless complications occur
(2) need to assess first
(3) *correct*—difficulty eating causes the CVA client severe anxiety
(4) positioning stipulations are not required unless complications occur

68. A client begins taking haloperidol (Haldol) 5 mg tid. It is MOST important for the nurse to make which of the following statements?

1. "Do not eat aged cheese, beer, or red wine."
2. "Rise slowly when standing."
3. "Suck on hard candy."
4. "Avoid pretzels, potato chips, and carbonated beverages."

Strategy: All answers are implementations. Determine the outcome of each answer. Is it desired?

(1) appropriate for a monoamine oxidase (MAO) inhibitor
(2) *correct*—side effect of Haldol is hypotension; moving slowly to a standing position will decrease the problem with orthostatic hypotension
(3) medication does not have anticholinergic effects
(4) salt does not have any effect on the medication

69. A nursing student with a history of breast cancer reports that she has just developed shingles on her trunk. Which of the following actions by the nurse is BEST?

1. Suggest that the nursing student contact her physician.
2. Assign the nursing student to clients that are not high risk.
3. Inform the nursing student that she cannot care for clients.
4. Restrict the nursing student from performing invasive procedures.

Strategy: Topic of the question is unstated. Read answer choices to determine topic.

(1) passing the buck; care of clients determined by the RN

(2) can't care for any clients until lesions have crusted

(3) *correct*—because student is immunocompromised, restrict from patient contact until lesions have crusted

(4) restricted from any patient contact

70. The nurse explains the use of transcutaneous electrical nerve stimulation (TENS) to a client with sciatica. Which of the following actions, if performed by the patient, would indicate that further teaching is necessary?

1. The client applies a conducting gel before applying the electrodes.
2. Client places the electrodes on the side of the body opposite to the painful area.
3. The client turns up the voltage until s/he feels a prickly "pins and needles" sensation.
4. The client adjusts the voltage based on the relief of pain s/he experiences.

Strategy: "Further teaching" indicates an in *correct* response.

(1) gel is used; should rotate sites to prevent irritation of skin

(2) *correct*—should be over, above, or below the painful area

(3) uses battery-operated device to deliver small currents to skin and underlying tissues

(4) used for localized pain, such as low back pain

71. The family members of an 85-year-old report to the nurse that they suspect that their father is masturbating. Which of the following responses by the nurse is BEST?

1. "I understand your concern because this is not a normal part of aging."
2. "Don't worry because I think that he will stop soon."
3. "This is considered a normal behavior for men."
4. "The best thing you can do is talk to your father about this behavior."

Strategy: Remember therapeutic communication.
(1) inappropriate
(2) inappropriate
(3) *correct*—masturbation is an activity performed by some elderly men
(4) would embarrass the father and cause him to have feelings of guilt and anxiety

72. A client has an order for aminophylline PO. The nurse should withhold the medication and notify the physician if the client makes which of the following statements?

1. "I am allergic to Neomycin."
2. "I am taking Isuprel."
3. "I have trouble breathing when I exercise."
4. "I have had several urinary tract infections."

Strategy: Determine the significance of each answer choice and how it relates to aminophylline.
(1) aminoglycosides are antibiotics
(2) *correct*—order for aminophylline should be questioned and/or verified for clients with a history of preexisting cardiac dysrhythmia
(3) medication is given to treat airway problems
(4) urinary tract infections are not a concern

73. During the initial prenatal visit, the physician orders an iron supplement to be taken throughout the client's pregnancy. It would be MOST important for the nurse to include which of the following instructions?"

1. "The medication should be taken with orange juice."

2. "Take the medication with antacids to decrease gastric distress."

3. "Drinking eight ounces of water will enhance absorption of the medication."

4. "Notify the physician if your stools become dark or loose."

Strategy: All answers are implementations. Determine the outcome of each answer choice. Is it desired?

(1) *correct*—vitamin C facilitates absorption of iron

(2) antacids will decrease absorption of the iron

(3) client needs increased fluids; fluids will not affect absorption

(4) stools will turn dark, but there is no need to notify the doctor

74. A client who had an appendectomy 4 days ago complains of severe abdominal pain. During the initial assessment he states, "I have had two almost-black stools today." Which of the following nursing actions is MOST important?

1. Start an IV with D5W at 125 cc/h.

2. Insert a nasogastric tube.

3. Notify the physician.

4. Obtain a stool specimen.

Strategy: All answers are implementations. Determine the outcome of each answer choice. Is it desired?

(1) requires a physician's order and would probably be ordered after the nurse notified the doctor of the findings

(2) requires a physician's order and would probably be ordered after the nurse notified the doctor of the findings

(3) *correct*—development of black, tarry stool in the presence of abdominal pain could represent gastrointestinal bleeding; should be reported to physician as soon as possible

(4) requires a physician's order and would probably be ordered after the nurse notified the doctor of the findings

75. The parents of a child who has just been diagnosed with a chronic illness share with the nurse that they are concerned about the sibling's sudden change in behavior. Which of the following is the BEST response by the nurse?

1. "Her brother is feeling left out right now, but we plan to include him in his sister's care."
2. "Her brother is just feeling left out right now, but will start acting normal soon."
3. "Her brother is worried about her and is just reacting to his fear."
4. "Her brother is going through a normal developmental stage."

Strategy: Answers are implementations. Determine the outcome of each answer choice. Is it desired?

(1) *correct*—total family participation is accomplished when you include the sibling
(2) appropriate, but does not help the family adjust to a child with a chronic illness
(3) appropriate, but does not help the family adjust to a child with a chronic illness
(4) inaccurate

76. The nurse is caring for a patient following a right adrenalectomy. During the immediate postoperative period, it is MOST important for the nurse to observe for which of the following?

1. Fluid and electrolyte imbalance.
2. Temperature fluctuation.
3. Respiratory atelectasis.
4. Blood pressure alteration.

Strategy: Remember the ABCs.

(1) severity of this complication is not as life-threatening as that of shock
(2) severity of this complication is not as life-threatening as that of shock
(3) severity of this complication is not as life-threatening as that of shock
(4) *correct*—decrease in blood pressure may indicate shock

77. A client on continuous mechanical ventilation desires to go home. In order to determine the client's ability for homecare, the nurse should

1. assess the ability of others in the home to be trained to provide appropriate care for the client.
2. confer with the client's physician and discuss the feasibility of the client's request.
3. assess the number of people in the home and the adequacy of space to care for the client.
4. examine the client's reasons for wanting to go home, and discuss the implications of homecare.

Strategy: Determine how the assessment relates to homecare.
(1) *correct*—to ensure safety and to provide client with quality care at home, assessing ability of others in home is critical before proceeding with efforts to discharge the client
(2) should occur, but ensuring that someone can care for the client should occur before consulting with the physician
(3) may be appropriate after the home situation is evaluated
(4) may occur, but first determine if someone can care for the client

78. Prior to helping a client out of bed on the first day after an anterior cervical fusion, the nurse should

1. remove the client's cervical collar.
2. raise the head of the bed.
3. position the client supine at the edge of the bed.
4. ask the client to fold both arms across his chest.

Strategy: All answers are implementations. Determine the outcome of each answer choice. Is it desired?
(1) contraindicated; collar offers additional support for the neck
(2) *correct*—raising head of bed decreases the effort for the client and the nurse
(3) inconvenient and would cause undue strain on the client
(4) does not allow the client to assist in the transfer

79. The daughter of an 80-year-old woman with Alzheimer's disease provides care for her mother in her home. The nurse knows that which of the following observations would most likely represent caregiver burnout?

1. The daughter fails to get her mother into a wheelchair daily.
2. The home environment is extremely cluttered at each visit.
3. The daughter is always in a housecoat at the times of the visits.
4. The daughter's husband is seen assisting with his mother-in-law's care.

Strategy: Think about what the words mean. How do they relate to the caregiver?
(1) may be impossible for the daughter to do alone
(2) *correct*—cluttered environment may represent depression and burnout
(3) may reveal the limited time the daughter has to take care of herself
(4) is very healthy and desirable

80. The nurse assesses the daily lab reports for a patient with a long history of cirrhosis with acute hepatic encephalopathy. Which of the following findings would indicate to the nurse that the patient is improving?

1. The patient's fasting blood sugar decreased from 100 to 90 mg/dL.
2. The patient's prothrombin time (PT) increased from 20 to 25 seconds.
3. The patient's ammonia level decreased from 160 to 120 mg/dL.
4. The patient's AST (SGOT) increased from 24 to 30 units.

Strategy: Determine the significance of each assessment and how it relates to hepatic encephalopathy.
(1) normal FBS 70–120 mg/dL, indicates glucose metabolism; usually altered with diabetes
(2) normal PT 11–15 seconds, indicates blood coagulation; usually altered with cirrhosis or anticoagulant medications, would decrease if improving
(3) *correct*—indicates a decrease in ammonia, normal ammonia 80–110 mg/dL
(4) normal 8–20 units, indicates liver damage; usually altered with acute pancreatitis and cirrhosis, indicates increased hepatic cell damage

81. When using palpation techniques during the physical assessment of an adult female with abdominal pain, which of the following actions should the nurse take FIRST?

1. Instruct the client to take a deep breath and hold it.
2. Inform the client to breathe slowly.
3. Use bimanual palpation technique.
4. Apply light palpation in the area.

Strategy: All answers are implementations. Determine the outcome of each answer choice. Is it desired?

(1) holding a deep breath is done during palpation of the liver

(2) *correct*—breathing slowly will enhance relaxation of the abdominal muscles

(3) bimanual palpation shouldn't be used for a client with abdominal pain

(4) prior to the abdominal palpation, instruct client to breathe slowly because client likely to protect the abdomen when in pain

82. Which of the following interventions should be the priority during the nursing care of a two-monthold infant after surgery?

1. Minimize stimuli for the infant.
2. Restrain all of the infant's extremities.
3. Encourage the parents to stroke the infant.
4. Demonstrate to the parents how they can assist with their infant's care.

Strategy: Answers are implementations. Determine the outcome of each answer choice. Is it desired?

(1) would lead to further deprivation

(2) would lead to further deprivation

(3) *correct*—tactile stimulation is imperative for an infant's normal emotional development; after
the trauma of surgery, sensory deprivation can cause failure to thrive

(4) does not address the emotional needs of the infant

83. On the morning after surgery to repair a fractured hip, the nurse finds a 66-year-old woman struggling to get out of bed. The client tells the nurse, "I have to clean the kitchen now." Which of the following actions, if taken by the nurse, is MOST appropriate?

1. Obtain blood gas studies.
2. Instruct the client to remain in bed.
3. Take the client's blood pressure.
4. Ask the family to remain with the client.

Strategy: Answers are a mix of assessments and implementations. Does this situation require assessment? Yes. Is there an appropriate assessment? Yes.

(1) *correct*—assessment; fat embolism is common with fractures of long bones, results in pulmonary or cerebral emboli, interferes with adequate circulation, confusion is first symptom
(2) need to assess first
(3) assessment; need to obtain ABG, start oxygen
(4) implementation; doesn't address the fat embolism

84. The nursing team includes three RNs, one LPN/LVN, and one nursing assistant. The nurse should consider the assignments appropriate if the nursing assistant is assigned to which of the following clients?

1. A client with an appendectomy.
2. A client with infectious meningitis.
3. An immunosuppressed client.
4. A client who had a radical mastectomy.

Strategy: RN cannot delegate clients that require assessment, teaching, or nursing judgment.

(1) *correct*—stable client with standard, unchanging procedures
(2) requires assessment; RN should care for this client
(3) requires skills of RN
(4) requires assessment and teaching

85. The nurse reading an EKG rhythm strip determines that there are 8 QRS complexes in 30 large squares for a 6-second strip. The nurse calculates the heart rate to be which of the following?

1. 60.
2. 70.
3. 80.
4. 120.

Strategy: Do the math.
(1) inaccurate
(2) inaccurate
(3) *correct*—30 large squares on the EKG paper represent six seconds; multiply the number of QRS complexes found in 30 large squares by ten (8 10 = 80 beats per minute)
(4) inaccurate

86. After abdominal surgery, a client complains of gas pains in her abdomen. It is MOST important for the nurse to take which of the following actions?

1. Offer the client fresh fruits and vegetables.
2. Ambulate the client frequently.
3. Teach the client how to splint the abdomen during activity.
4. Position the client on her right side.

Strategy: All answers are implementations. Determine the outcome of each answer choice. Is it desired?
(1) Not encouraged until the bowel sounds returned and client is able to eat, will help prevent constipation, but will not prevent gas pains
(2) *correct*—ambulation promotes active peristalsis, facilitates expulsion of flatus
(3) does nothing to increase peristalsis, which is needed after surgery
(4) does nothing to increase peristalsis, which is needed after surgery

87. A client has recently been placed on warfarin (Coumadin) for transient ischemic attacks (TIAs). The nurse would be MOST concerned if the patient made which of the following statements?

1. "I eat cantaloupe and bananas every day."
2. "I can eat potato chips and dill pickles."
3. "I eat strawberries and oranges every day."
4. "I have to eat more green salads and pork."

Strategy: Determine the nutrients contained in each answer and how they relate to Coumadin.

(1) high in potassium; would have no effect on the medication

(2) high in sodium; would have no effect on the medication

(3) high in vitamin C; would have no effect on the medication

(4) *correct*—ingestion of large quantities of foods high in vitamin K content may antagonize the anticoagulant effect of warfarin

88. A 34-year-old man is seen in the physician's office for follow-up after treatment for renal calculi. The nurse discusses methods to prevent a reoccurrence of the problem. Which of the following instructions by the nurse is MOST beneficial?

1. "Drink at least 3,000 ml of fluid a day."
2. "Reduce the amount of dairy products and eggs in your diet."
3. "Increase the amount of whole grains and vegetables you eat."
4. "Avoid foods that contain tyramine, such as wine and cheese."

Strategy: "MOST beneficial" indicates priority. All answers are implementations. Determine the outcome of each answer choice. Is it desired?

(1) *correct*—prevention program: diet, medications, fluids 3,000 to 4,000 ml/day

(2) only helpful if known composition of stones; information not presented

(3) dietary changes helpful if composition of stones known

(4) should be avoided if taking MAO-inhibitor medications such as Marplan to treat depression

89. The nurse is observing the psychiatric staff interact with a client exhibiting manipulative behavior. The nurse should intervene in which of the following situations?

1. The staff discusses with the client the consequences of the manipulative behavior.
2. The staff collaborates to establish limits on the manipulative behavior.
3. The staff clarifies the consequences of the client's manipulative behavior.
4. The staff decreases demands placed on the client that triggers the manipulative behavior.

Strategy: "The nurse would intervene" means you are looking for an in_correct_ **response.**
(1) appropriate and effective strategy for intervening with a manipulative client
(2) appropriate and effective strategy for intervening with a manipulative client
(3) appropriate and effective strategy for intervening with a manipulative client
(4) *correct*—can foster a sense of entitlement along with underfunctioning; establishing realistic, achievable goals and activities is necessary to build self-esteem

90. A 32-year-old male with acute lymphocytic leukemia is admitted with shortness of breath, anemia, and tachycardia. The MOST appropriately stated nursing diagnosis would be

1. Altered protection, immunosuppression: leukemia.
2. Impaired gas exchange related to decreased RBCs.
3. Risk for infection related to altered immune system.
4. Risk of injury related to decreased platelets.

Strategy: Think about each answer choice.
(1) incorrectly stated
(2) *correct*—leukemia causes a decrease in all blood components; a gas exchange problem results from depletion of oxygen-carrying red cells
(3) relates to leukemia, but does not support the assessment data in the question
(4) relates to leukemia, but does not support the assessment data in the question

91. An order has been received to obtain a stool specimen and test for occult blood. The nurse would be MOST concerned if the client made which of the following statements?

1. "I take Feosol every day."
2. "My physician prescribed Vicodin."
3. "I've been taking Lomotil."
4. "I sometimes take Motrin."

Strategy: Determine the action of each drug and how it relates to a stool specimen.

(1) *correct*—iron supplements can cause color of stool to resemble melena
(2) opiate narcotic; would have little effect on stool specimen reliability
(3) antidiarrheal; would have little effect on stool specimen reliability
(4) nonsteroidal antiinflammatory drug (NSAID); would have little effect on stool specimen
reliability

92. A 60-year-old woman receives thiethylperazine maleate (Torecan) 10 mg IM after surgery for repair of a hernia. The ordered activity is up ad lib. One half-hour after administration of the medication, the patient has to void. The nurse should

1. accompany the patient to the bathroom.
2. place the patient on the bedpan.
3. obtain a bedside commode for the patient to use.
4. obtain an order to catheterize the patient.

Strategy: All answers are implementations. Determine the outcome of each answer choice. Is it desired?

(1) stay in bed 1 hour after getting medication, possible orthostatic hypotension
(2) *correct*—necessary for patient safety
(3) stay in bed 1 hour after getting medication, possible orthostatic hypotension
(4) unnecessary invasive procedure

93. The nurse is caring for a client recovering from lower bowel surgery. The nurse determines that teaching has been successful if the client selects which of the following menus?

1. Milk, green beans, whole-wheat bread.
2. Creamed chicken soup, broccoli, pudding.
3. Baked chicken, buttered rice, plain gelatin.
4. Cabbage salad, fried chicken, applesauce.

Strategy: Determine what type of diet is required. Select the menu that reflects the diet.

(1) contains a high-residue food

(2) contains a high-residue food

(3) *correct*—low-residue diet will leave a relatively small amount of residue, or indigestible material, in the colon; all meats, fish, and poultry must be broiled or baked

(4) contains a high-residue food

94. The nurse is caring for a teenaged boy in Buck's traction. It is MOST important for the nurse to take which of the following actions?

1. Check the pin sites for bleeding or infection.
2. Apply topical or antibiotic ointment as ordered.
3. Assess that the elastic bandages are not too loose or too tight.
4. Remove the bandages daily to lubricate the skin.

Strategy: Answers are a mix of assessments and implementations. Is the assessment appropriate? Yes.

(1) Buck's traction is a type of skin traction; there are no pins

(2) Buck's traction is a type of skin traction; there is no need for topical ointment

(3) *correct*—nurse needs to assess the client to make sure circulation is not being compromised

(4) skin is not lubricated under the bandages

95. A 41-year-old woman was brought to the emergency room by two police officers after she had been standing barefoot in the rain for more than two hours. The police officers report that the woman had to be restrained after she resisted and became agitated. The intake nurse's FIRST action should be to

1. complete a physical examination.
2. maintain a safe environment.
3. ascertain the client's mental status.
4. orient the client to place and time.

Strategy: Answers are a mix of assessments and implementations. Does this situation require validation? No. Determine the best implementation.

(1) assessment; should not be first action

(2) *correct*—implementation; major priority of the nurse is to provide and maintain safety for the client who is unable to provide for herself; safe environment will generate trust and rapport; will decrease resistance to doing preliminary physical exam, which includes orienting client and doing a mental status exam

(3) assessment; should not be first action

(4) implementation; should not be first action

96. A nursing team consists of an RN, an LPN/LVN, and a nursing assistant. The nurse should assign which of the following patients to the LPN/LVN?

1. A 72-year-old patient with diabetes who requires a dressing change for a stasis ulcer.
2. A 55-year-old patient with terminal cancer being transferred to hospice homecare.
3. A 42-year-old patient with cancer of the bone complaining of pain.
4. A 23-year-old patient with a fracture of the right leg who asks to use the urinal.

Strategy: Think about the skill level involved in each patient's care.

(1) *correct*—stable patient with an expected outcome

(2) requires nursing judgment; RN is the appropriate caregiver

(3) requires assessment; RN is the appropriate caregiver

(4) standard unchanging procedure; assign to the nursing assistant

97. A primipara is admitted in early labor, and her membranes rupture. Which of the following assessments by the nurse is MOST important?

1. Determine the pH of the amniotic fluid.
2. Evaluate the mother's blood pressure.
3. Check the monitor for decelerations.
4. Assess for a prolapsed cord.

Strategy: Determine how each answer choice relates to the rupture of membranes.

(1) amniotic fluid is important to check to differentiate it from urine; pH will be acidic if it is urine

(2) mother's blood pressure is not affected by rupture of the membranes

(3) nurse should look for variable decelerations if cord is prolapsed

(4) *correct*—initial assessment is to check for a prolapsed cord

98. A client had a mitral valve replacement three days ago. It is MOST important for the nurse to take which of the following actions?

1. Maintain the client in the supine position to prevent tension on the mediastinal suture line.
2. Encourage deep breathing, but discourage coughing because of increased central venous pressure.
3. Decrease fluids to prevent fluid retention and development of congestive heart failure.
4. Encourage early activity to promote ventilation and improve quality of circulation.

Strategy: All answers are implementations. Determine the outcome of each answer choice. Is it desired?

(1) client is maintained in semi-Fowler's position

(2) coughing and deep breathing should be encouraged

(3) fluids are encouraged unless there is evidence of cardiac failure

(4) *correct*—postoperative open heart clients should be out of bed and ambulating as soon as possible, frequently one to two days after surgery

99. The physician orders an arterial blood gas (ABG) for a client receiving oxygen at 6 L/min. Results show: pH 7.37, HCO3 26 mEq/L, pCO2 42 mm Hg, pO2 90 mm Hg. The nurse should

1. increase the rate of oxygen flow the patient is receiving.
2. elevate the head of the bed.
3. document the results in the chart.
4. instruct the patient to cough and deep breathe.

Strategy: All answers are implementations. Determine the outcome of each answer choice. Is it desired?

(1) oxygen level normal
(2) unnecessary, results normal
(3) *correct*—results normal, should be recorded
(4) unnecessary, results normal

100. A client is given an aminophylline (Somophyllin) capsule four hours too early. This incident is discovered 30 minutes after administration of the medication. The nurse should

1. document the event on an incident report form and notify the physician.
2. change the time for the next medication administration.
3. assess for bradycardia and lethargy and notify the physician.
4. skip the next dose of the medication.

Strategy: All answers are implementations. Determine the outcome of each answer choice. Is it desired?

(1) *correct*—documenting the error on an incident report, assessing for side effects, and
notifying the physician would be the most appropriate actions for the nurse to take
(2) unsafe, in *correct* nursing intervention
(3) unsafe, in *correct* nursing intervention
(4) unsafe, in *correct* nursing intervention

101. A pregnant client at 16-weeks gestation has a blood sample for rubella antibody screening drawn. The test results reveal a low titer. When discussing the results with the client, the nurse should

1. arrange for her to have an MMR immunization immediately.

2. explain to her that the results are expected and nothing needs to be done.

3. explore options with her about whether or not she should terminate the pregnancy.

4. encourage her to receive the rubella immunization immediately after delivery.

Strategy: Answers are implementations. Determine the outcome of each answer choice. Is it desired?

(1) active immunization should not be administered

(2) should not be done in this situation

(3) should not be done in this situation

(4) *correct*—with a low rubella titer, the client is at risk for developing rubella; immediately after delivery, within early postpartum period she needs to receive an immunization

102. The nurse is caring for a patient with a head injury. Appropriate nursing interventions for minimizing the risk of increasing intracranial pressure include

1. maintaining a liquid diet, performing frequent tracheal suctioning, and turning the client every two hours.

2. keeping the head of the bed flat, turning the client every two hours, and performing nasotracheal suctioning every hour.

3. maintaining the head of the bed elevated at 90°, keeping the room dark and quiet, and placing the call light within easy reach.

4. keeping the patient's head from flexing or rotating, elevating the head of the bed 30°, and avoiding frequent suctioning for more than 15 seconds.

Strategy: All answers are implementations. Determine the outcome of each answer choice. Is it desired?

(1) tracheal suctioning should be done only as necessary because it will increase intracranial pressure

(2) tracheal suctioning should be done only as necessary because it will increase intracranial pressure

(3) is appropriate only if client is awake and alert

(4) *correct*—objective is to increase venous return and decrease cerebral edema

103. The nurse is preparing to discharge a woman after an abdominal cholecystectomy for treatment of cholelithiasis. The nurse should tell the woman to contact her physician if

1. her sleeping pattern changes from before surgery.
2. her bowel movements become soft and tan in color.
3. her tolerance for fatty foods increases.
4. she voids five times a day and her urine is pale yellow.

Strategy: Determine how each answer choice relates to biliary obstruction

(1) unnecessary to notify the physician
(2) *correct*—indicates biliary obstruction; bile pigments needed to color stool dark brown color
(3) unnecessary to call physician; individual tolerance for foods vary
(4) normal voiding pattern

104. A 43 year-old man has been receiving cimetidine (Tagamet) 300 mg qid for several weeks. During an office visit the physician gives him an additional prescription for aluminum hydroxide (Amphojel) 600 mg qid. Which of the following instructions, if given by the nurse, is BEST?

1. Tagamet and Amphojel together after meals and hs for combined effect.
2. Amphojel with meals and before bed and Tagamet 1 h after meals and before bed.
3. Take the Tagamet 2 h before meals and before bed and the Amphojel 2 h after meals and at bedtime.
4. Tagamet with meals and 1 h before bed, Amphojel 2 h after meals,hs.

Strategy: All answers are implementations. Determine the outcome of each answer choice. Is it desired?

(1) antacids interfere with absorption of Tagamet, should be separated by 1 h
(2) Amphojel should be given 1 h after meals and Tagamet with meals
(3) Tagamet should be given with meals and Amphojel 1 h after meals
(4) *correct*—give Tagamet with meals (causes more consistent therapeutic effect) and hs, antacids interfere with absorption, separate administration by 1 h, give Amphojel 1 hr after meals and hs

105. The nurse is caring for a patient the second day after an appendectomy. The patient is a 23 year-old exchange student from Japan. Which of the following observations by the nurse would suggest that the patient is experiencing pain?

1. The patient's pulse is 74, BP 104/66.
2. The patient's dressing has a small amount of serosanguinous drainage.
3. The patient repeatedly rubs his hands together.
4. The patient's skin is cool and dry.

Strategy: Determine how each answer choice relates to pain.

(1) would expect BP and pulse to increase in response to pain

(2) no relationship with drainage from incision and pain

(3) *correct*—nurse should assess for nonverbal cues to pain, such as increased confusion, restlessness, aggressive behaviors

(4) would expect patient to be diaphoretic in response to pain

106. Client complains 3 days after above-knee amputation (AKA), about phantom limb pain in his lower leg. Which is nursing responses is BEST?

1. "That should improve within a year."
2. "I'll call the physician."
3. "Keep your leg on this pillow."
4. "Staying active will help decrease the episodes."

Strategy: All answers are implementations. Determine the outcome of each answer choice. Is it desired?

(1) may be true for 2% of amputees, but for the majority, pain occurs for a few months

(2) passing the buck

(3) contraindicated after 24 hours because of possibility of causing contractures

(4) *correct*—activity helps reduce frequency and degree of phantom pain

107. The nurse is observing care given to a client who vigorously follows several rituals daily, including frequent handwashing. The client's hands are now reddened and sensitive to touch. The nurse should intervene if which of the following is observed?

1. The staff administers special skin care to the client.
2. The staff gives positive reinforcement for nonritualistic behavior.
3. The staff limits the amount of time the client may use to wash hands.
4. The staff protects the client from ridicule by other clients on the unit.

Strategy: "Should intervene" indicates that you are looking for in *correct* behavior. Don't lose the question.
(1) appropriate nursing action
(2) appropriate nursing action
(3) *correct*—will only increase the client's anxiety and need for the rituals, limits must be
gradually instituted
(4) appropriate nursing action

108. An elderly man is constantly coming to the nurse's station with varying complaints and requests. Which is the nurse is BEST?

1. Speak to him only when called by him.
2. Address and manage each specific complaint and request.
3. Redirect him to other activity.
4. See him at consistent intervals, even when not complaining or requesting it.

Strategy: All answers are implementations. Determine the outcome of each answer choice. Is it desired?
(1) can escalate his feelings of abandonment
(2) not the best action, and would not serve to reduce the behavior
(3) can escalate his feelings of abandonment
(4) *correct*—client is probably fearful of being abandoned; interacting with the client at consistent intervals when he is not complaining will begin to reduce the calling, requesting, and complaining behaviors

109. The physician prescribes estrogen (Premarin) 0.625 mg daily for a 43-year-old woman. Which of the following statements, if made by the client to the nurse, indicates that further teaching is necessary?

1. "There may be a change in my libido due to this medication."
2. "I may have a change in my weight while taking this medication."
3. "I may have some difficulty wearing my contact lenses because of the medication."
4. "It is unnecessary for me to perform routine self-breast exams while I am taking this medication."

Strategy: "Further teaching is necessary" indicates that you are looking for wrong information.
(1) common side effects
(2) common side effect
(3) causes dryness of eyes
(4) *correct*—should continue to perform monthly self-breast exams

110. Which of the following statements made to the nurse by a mother who is breastfeeding indicates a need for further teaching?

1. "I will go to my doctor and get fitted for a diaphragm."
2. "I will ask my husband use a condom."
3. "I will get a prescription from my doctor for the Pill."
4. "I will practice abstinence during my fertile time."

Strategy: Topic of question is unstated. Read answer choices for clues.
(1) could be used and does not indicate a need for further teaching
(2) could be used and does not indicate a need for further teaching
(3) *correct*—the Pill (oral contraceptive) suppresses production of breast milk; while breastfeeding, another method of contraception should be used
(4) could be used and does not indicate a need for further teaching

111. A 19-year-old client is seen in the emergency room for an overdose of acetylsalicylic acid (aspirin). Which of the following actions by the nurse is BEST?

1. Determine when the client took the aspirin.
2. Initiate an intravenous infusion and administer protamine sulfate.
3. Administer Vitamin K (AquaMEPHYTON).
4. Obtain an arterial blood gas and request respiratory therapy to begin respiratory support.

Strategy: Answers are a mix of assessments and implementations. Is assessment required? Yes. Is there an appropriate assessment? Yes.

(1) *correct*—charcoal, if given within two hours, will absorb particles of salicylate
(2) antidote for heparin
(3) antidote for warfarin (Coumadin)
(4) may be necessary later, but current need is to evaluate response to charcoal

112. The nurse is evaluating care given to clients by the home health aide. The nurse would intervene in which of the following situations?

1. The nursing assistant walks a client 15 feet with a walker.
2. The nursing assistant feeds a blind client using a spoon.
3. The nursing assistant administers a client's medication.
4. The nursing assistant performs catheter care for a client.

Strategy: "Nurse would intervene" indicates an in *correct* action.
(1) appropriate action; standard, unchanging procedure
(2) appropriate action; standard, unchanging procedure
(3) *correct*—care not within the scope of a nursing assistant
(4) appropriate action

113. The nurse is caring for a patient who has been lethargic but responsive to verbal commands. The nurse now observes that the client is responding to noxious stimuli by withdrawing. The MOST appropriate nursing action is to:

1. reassess the client in one hour.
2. notify the physician.
3. place the client in Trendelenburg position.
4. contact the family.

Strategy: Answers are a mix of assessments and implementations. Does this situation require validation? No. Determine the outcome of the implementations.

(1) validation not required

(2) *correct*—withdrawing from pain is a sign of deterioration in client's condition; doctor should be notified

(3) will increase the cranial pressure

(4) physician should be notified immediately

114. A 62-year-old man is undergoing peritoneal dialysis at a hemodialysis center. The nurse notices that the fluid outflow is inadequate. Which of the following activities, if performed by the nurse, would be best INITIALLY?

1. Place the man in low-Fowler's position.
2. Position the drainage bag at the level of the man's heart.
3. Close the clamp to the drainage tubing for one-half hour, and then reopen.
4. Milk the drainage tubing firmly every 20 minutes.

Strategy: All answers are implementations. Determine the outcome of each answer choice. Is it desired?

(1) *correct*—minimizes the build-up of intra-abdominal pressure

(2) should be lower than patient's abdomen to allow for drainage by gravity

(3) all clamps should be open

(4) not best first action; done carefully as needed if fibrin clot has formed

115. A 36-year-old woman is being treated for rheumatoid arthritis. Which of the following findings should assume the HIGHEST priority for the nurse when planning her care?

1. The woman has subcutaneous nodules on her right and left forearms.
2. The woman has a slight contracture of her right wrist.
3. The woman has mild erythema of her finger joints.
4. The woman has an area of ecchymosis approximately 3 mm in diameter on right forearm.

Strategy: Determine the significance of each answer choice and how it relates to rheumatoid arthritis.

(1) expected symptom of disease

(2) *correct*—sign of inadequate management; should be treated immediately to prevent further damage

(3) redness expected symptom of disease

(4) may be results of mild trauma, not highest priority

116. The nurse is evaluating care for a client with depression. The nurse would be MOST concerned if which of the following was observed?

1. The LPN/LVN teaches the client deep breathing and relaxation techniques.
2. The staff allows the client to verbalize what he is thinking when he tries to sleep.
3. The staff encourages the client to express his feelings more clearly.
4. The LPN/LVN administers flurazepam hydrochloride (Dalmane) 15 mg hs.

Strategy: "MOST concerned" indicates an in *correct* action.

(1) therapeutic intervention to help the client learn how to create an environment conducive to sleep

(2) therapeutic intervention to help the client learn how to create an environment conducive to sleep

(3) therapeutic intervention to help the client learn how to create an environment conducive to sleep

(4) *correct*—medication that produces dependence should be a last resort; used only if other nursing measures and antidepressant medications have not worked and the client is exhausted

117. A permanent demand pacemaker, set at a rate of 72, is implanted in a client for persistent thirddegree block. The nurse would be MOST concerned if which of the following was observed?

1. Pulse rate 88 and irregular.
2. Apical pulse rate regular at 68.
3. Blood pressure 110/88, pulse at 78.
4. Skin warm and dry to touch.

Strategy: Determine how each answer relates to a pacemaker.
(1) does not indicate malfunction of the pacemaker
(2) *correct*—any time the pulse rate drops below the preset rate on the pacemaker, the pacer is malfunctioning; the pulse should be maintained at a minimal rate set on the pacemaker
(3) does not indicate malfunction of the pacemaker
(4) may be an early sign of infection at the site

118. A mother tells you that the seven-year-old sibling of her child with cystic fibrosis is having difficulty in school, fights frequently with playmates, and throws his toys. Which of the following would be the BEST response by the nurse?

1. "Did he have these behaviors before his sister was diagnosed?"
2. "That is typical of seven-year-olds."
3. "Spend time with each child daily, and it will stop."
4. "He is jealous of the attention his sister is receiving."

Strategy: Answers are a mix of assessments and implementations. Does this situation require assessment? Yes. Is there an appropriate assessment? Yes.
(1) *correct*—assess for a cause of the disruptive behavior
(2) dismisses parent's concern
(3) implementation; nurse must assess behavior prior to his sibling's illness
(4) nurse must assess behavior prior to his sibling's illness

119. The nurse is admitting a client with possible Haemophilus influenzae—meningitis. It is MOST important for the nurse to take which of the following actions?

1. Place the client on airborne precautions for twenty-four hours.
2. Perform neurological checks every four to six hours.
3. Dim the lights in the room and minimize environmental stimuli.
4. Encourage PO fluids during the day to decrease fever.

Strategy: Answers are a mix of assessments and implementations. Is the assessment appropriate? No. Determine the outcome of implementations.
(1) implementation; clients with meningitis are placed on droplet for at least 24 hours
(2) assessment; although these assessments are important, they should be done more frequently
(3) *correct*—implementation; will minimize the likelihood of seizures
(4) implementation; fluid restriction due to increased intracranial pressure

120. The nurse prepares a 56-year-old woman for insertion of a subclavian triple lumen catheter to be used for administration of total parenteral nutrition (TPN). The nurse should position the client

1. in high-Fowler's position with the client's head in a neutral position.
2. in semi-Fowler's position with the client's head extended.
3. supine with the client's head low and turned away from the insertion site.
4. left lateral with the client's head turned toward the insertion site.

Strategy: All answers are implementations. Determine the outcome of each answer choice. Is it desired?
(1) would not promote dilation of blood vessels involved
(2) would not promote dilation of blood vessels involved
(3) *correct*—produces dilation of neck and shoulder vessels, making entry easier and preventing air embolus
(4) not best position; client should turn head away for insertion site

121. The nurse is obtaining a health history from the mother of a child with failure to thrive. Which of the following assessments would provide the MOST pertinent data?

1. Weight and height.
2. Urine output.
3. Type of feedings.
4. Mother/child interactions.

Strategy: Determine how each answer choice relates to failure to thrive.

(1) *correct*—physical, provides the most pertinent data in assessing actual growth
(2) physical; indicates hydration status
(3) physical; but not most important assessment
(4) psychosocial; physical takes priority

122. The nurse cares for a 44-year-old man in the clinic. The physician's orders read: sulindac (Clinoril) 200 mg PO bid for 14 days. The nurse should instruct the man to report which of the following symptoms IMMEDIATELY to the physician?

1. Nervousness.
2. Photophobia.
3. Ecchymosis of the extremities.
4. Slight edema of the feet.

Strategy: Determine the cause of each answer and how it relates to Clinoril.

(1) side effect, but not most important
(2) not side effect
(3) *correct*—should notify physician if easy bruising or prolonged bleeding occurs
(4) does cause sodium retention, but not most important

123. The nurse is caring for clients in the prenatal clinic. The nurse would be MOST concerned if a diabetic client in the third trimester makes which of the following statements?

1. "I am taking less insulin now than I did two months ago."
2. "I am eating a large bedtime snack."
3. "I walk 15 minutes after lunch every day."
4. "I check my blood sugar two hours after each meal."

Strategy: "MOST concerned" indicates you are looking for a complication.

(1) *correct*—placenta produces hormones that make the cells insulin-resistant; as pregnancy progresses, these hormones increase; if insulin requirement is decreased, this indicates that the placenta is not functioning appropriately

(2) recommended to prevent hypoglycemia and starvation ketosis during the night

(3) best time for exercise is after meals when blood glucose is rising

(4) postprandial measurements done to prevent hyperglycemia; also check blood sugars before meals and at bedtime

124. Which of the following provides the best evidence that the nursing interventions to deal with a client's self-care deficit in relation to feeding have been effective?

1. The client eats at least one-half of all meals and drinks a minimum of 2,000 mL/day.
2. The client's dentures have been replaced, and he is able to chew.
3. The client will eat without verbalizing suspicions when a particular nurse sits with him.
4. The client appears to have increased energy to complete grooming activities.

Strategy: Determine the outcome of each answer choice. Is it desired?

(1) *correct*—concrete measure of the client's eating patterns indicates adequate intake of a well-balanced diet

(2) may not represent a well-balanced diet

(3) indicates the client is still experiencing distorted thinking about the foods he is to eat

(4) may not be an accurate measure of adequate nutrition

125. The nurse is working at a student health clinic at a large university. Which of the following signs and symptoms would cause the nurse to suspect cocaine abuse in a 20-year-old college student?

1. Frequent sneezing, complaints of a sore throat, and a temperature of 100°F (37.8°C).
2. Diarrhea, vomiting, and abdominal pain.
3. Fatigue, dilated pupils, and anorexia.
4. Complaints of insomnia, rhinorrhea, and facial pain.

Strategy: Determine how each answer choice relates to cocaine abuse.
(1) suggests viral infection or allergic rhinitis
(2) could indicate GI problem or substance withdrawal
(3) could indicate any type of substance abuse or other illness
(4) *correct*—associated with cocaine use by inhalation, nose is most common route for administration

126. The nursing team consists of an RN who has been practicing for 6 months, a LPN/LVN who has been practicing for 15 years, and a nursing assistant who has been caring for clients for 3 years. The RN should care for which of the following clients?

1. A client 1-day postoperative after an internal fixation of a fractured left femur.
2. A client receiving diltiazem (Cardizem) and phenytoin (Dilantin).
3. A client who is to receive 2 units of packed cells prior to an upper endoscopy procedure.
4. A client admitted yesterday with exhaustion and a diagnosis of acute bipolar disorder.

Strategy: The RN cares for clients that require assessment, teaching, and nursing judgment.
(1) care can be assigned to the nursing assistant; standard, unchanging procedure
(2) medication can be given by the LPN
(3) *correct*—requires the assessment and teaching skills of RN
(4) offer food and fluids, assign to LPN

127. An 8-year-old boy is brought to the physician's office by his mother. The mother is concerned because the boy has a fever, vomited twice, and slept all day yesterday with the curtains closed. The boy complains of headache, nausea, and has a temperature of 103°F (39.3°C). The nurse observes the boy has a petechial rash on the trunk of his body. Which of the following assessments would be MOST important for the nurse to perform?

1. Grasp the child's hands and ask him to squeeze the nurse's hands.
2. Stroke the plantar surface of the child's foot with a reflex hammer.
3. Gently flex the child's head and neck onto the chest.
4. Have the child stand with his eyes closed, his arms at his sides, and his feet and knees close together.

Strategy: "MOST important" indicates a priority question. All answer choices are assessments. Determine why you would perform each assessment and how it relates to the situation.

(1) check of grasp strength is a nonspecific neurological check
(2) normal response plantar flexion of toes (negative Babinski); dorsiflexion of great toe and fanning of other toes (positive Babinski) abnormal in child older than 2; indicates CNS disease, not indicated in this situation
(3) *correct*—Brudzinski reflex, positive response (flexion of the hips and knees) indicates meningeal irritation
(4) Romberg's sign, nonspecific, assesses equilibrium and cerebellar functions

128. The nurse is preparing to discharge a client after an abdominal cholecystectomy for treatment of cholelithiasis. The client will go home with a T-tube in place. Which of the following statements, if made by the client to the nurse, indicates a need for further teaching?

1. "It will be great to finally get home, take a shower, and wash my hair."
2. "If the amount of drainage increases over the next several days, I should call my physician."
3. "I can resume swimming laps three times a week at my health club."
4. "I will check the skin around the tube once a day to see how it is doing.".

Strategy: All answers are implementations. Determine the outcome of each answer choice. Is it desired?

(1) maintains personal hygiene

(2) increase in bile drainage is sign of obstruction, should continue to decrease

(3) *correct*—should avoid strenuous exercise and do not immerse T-tube in water

(4) should check for signs of inflammation

129. A 68-year-old man is diagnosed with myasthenia gravis. The nurse instructs the client about his disease. Which of the following statements, if made by the client to the nurse, indicates the need for further teaching?

1. "I should not drink alcoholic beverages."

2. "I should not go places that are crowded."

3. "I should try to stay calm."

4. "I should use my hot tub daily."

Strategy: "Need for further teaching" indicates you are looking for an in*correct* statement.

(1) should be avoided

(2) may cause infection

(3) emotional extremes can cause exacerbations

(4) *correct*—should avoid heat (sauna, hot tubs, sunbathing)

130. The nurse is the leader of a group of mentally retarded adults. The nurse instructs the group members to ignore another client whenever he interrupts others who are speaking. To evaluate the progress of this intervention, the nurse should

1. measure improvement by counting the number of times the client succeeds.

2. measure improvement by counting the number of interruptions.

3. assess the ability of the group to control the client's interruptions.

4. count the number of tokens and earned privileges given for interruptions.

Strategy: Determine the outcome of each answer choice. Think about what the words mean.

(1) *correct*—nurse leader will be able to measure improvement by counting the number of times the client succeeds in controlling his interruptions when others are speaking; tokens can be awarded for successes and then exchanged for privileges; they would not be given for continued interruptions; belonging to a group and being allowed to go to group sessions can be a reward for the members; power of group helps to decrease socially unacceptable behavior

131. The nurse is caring for a four-year-old child with a closed head injury. The nurse would be reassured by which of the following observations?

1. The child is able to state his name when asked who he is.
2. The child reaches for a stuffed animal brought from home.
3. The child maintains himself in opisthotonos.
4. The child withdraws from mildly painful stimuli.

Strategy: "Nurse would be reassured" indicates a positive outcome.
(1) *correct*—being able to state one's name demonstrates orientation to person, positive sign with head trauma
(2) an act that even a disoriented child may perform
(3) indicates meningeal irritation
(4) may be observed in the unconscious cli

132. The mother of a 10-year-old boy with IDDM (insulin-dependent diabetes mellitus) calls to discuss the child's self-monitoring blood glucose (SMBG) home readings. He is being tightly regulated with a combination of NPH and regular insulin before breakfast and supper. The past two mornings his blood sugar readings were 220 mg/dl and 210 mg/dL. The nurse should advise the mother to

1. continue with his medication regime.
2. check his blood sugar during the night.
3. give his NPH insulin later in the evening.
4. serve his bedtime snack earlier in the evening.

Strategy: Answers are a mix of assessments and implementations. Does this situation require validation? Yes.
(1) implementation; is showing hyperglycemia, should try to find reason and prevent problem
(2) *correct*—assessment; may be having rebound hyperglycemia (Somogyi effect) following hypoglycemia episode while sleeping
(3) implementation; assumes that blood sugar is elevated all night; don't take action until cause determined
(4) implementation; must first determine cause of elevated readings; physician could increase amount of bedtime snack to prevent Somogyi effect

133. Client is in the outpatient clinic. After instilling atropine sulfate (Isopto Atropine) eye drops, the nurse should instruct the client to

1. hold pressure on the inner canthus for one minute.
2. keep the eyes opened and blink frequently to disperse the medication.
3. roll the eyes in all directions to enhance the action of the medication.
4. close the eyes tightly to prevent leakage of the medication.

Strategy: All answers are implementations. Determine the outcome of each answer choice. Is it desired?

(1) *correct*—holding pressure on the inner canthus decreases the amount of medication absorbed systemically

(2) not relevant to this medication

(3) not relevant to this medication

(4) not relevant to this medication

134. A spica cast has been applied to a 14-month-old with developmental dysplasia of the hips. Which of the following would be MOST appropriate for the nurse to teach the parents?

1. Change diapers frequently to prevent cast soiling.
2. Inspect the skin around the cast.
3. Turn the client by using the abduction stabilizer bar.
4. Keep small toys out of the client's reach.

Strategy: Answers are a mix of assessments and implementations. Does this situation require assessment? Yes. Is there an appropriate assessment? Yes.

(1) implementation; appropriate

(2) *correct*—assessment; assess for skin breakdown; change client's position frequently to prevent skin breakdown

(3) implementation; inappropriate

(4) implementation; appropriate, but is not higher priority than answer choice #2

135. A client has been placed on phenelzine sulfate (Nardil) 11 mg PO daily to assist in treating her current depression. The nurse determines that teaching has been effective if the client makes which of the following statements?

1. "I will call my doctor and stop taking the medication if I begin to have severe headaches."
2. "I can drink wine, but I should avoid alcoholic beverages that contain high levels of alcohol."
3. "I know I am going to feel better in a couple of days. I am so glad I finally got some medication."
4. "I can take the over-the-counter (OTC) cold medications that contain pseudoephedrine."

Strategy: All answers are implementations. Determine the outcome of each answer choice. Is it desired?

(1) *correct*—medication is an MAO inhibitor; hypertensive crisis may be precipitated by foods containing tyramine; client should be taught to report problems associated with hypertension
(2) wine is contraindicated; it contains tyramine
(3) takes up to two weeks for the medication to be effective
(4) cold medications with pseudoephedrine are contraindicated due to possible hypertensive problems

136. An 82-year-old female client is diagnosed with a vitamin K deficiency due to dietary malabsorption. Which of the following is an appropriate nursing intervention for this client?

1. Encourage the client to remain in bed.
2. Carefully check the client's arm after taking her blood pressure.
3. Increase dietary intake of fruits and fiber.
4. Observe the client for signs of angina or cardiac dysrhythmia.

Strategy: Answers are a mix of assessments and implementations. Does this situation require assessment? Yes.
(1) implementation; remaining in bed does not decrease the potential for bleeding
(2) *correct*—assessment; observe for bruising of the arm after taking a blood pressure reading
(3) implementation; does not affect absorption of vitamin K
(4) assessment; inappropriate for vitamin K deficiency

137. A father brings his 15-month-old son to the well-baby clinic for a routine check-up. The father confides to the nurse that he is concerned that his son still crawls and does not walk. Which of the following responses, if made by the nurse to the father, is BEST?

1. "I will refer you to a pediatric specialist if he doesn't start walking soon."
2. "Have you noticed any signs of paralysis or weakness in your son?"
3. "Try standing him on his feet several times a day."
4. "Children frequently set their own pace for development."

Strategy: "BEST" indicates priority.

(1) child usually begins walking 12–15 months of age, no reason for referral

(2) does not recognize behavior as normal

(3) children will walk when they are ready

(4) *correct*—children are individuals

138. A 45-year-old woman with hepatitis B is scheduled for an abdominal hysterectomy. It is MOST important for the nurse to check which of the following lab results before the patient goes to surgery?

1. Potassium.
2. Sodium.
3. Prothrombin time.
4. Hemoglobin.

Strategy: "MOST important" indicates a priority question. Determine what each value is measuring and how it relates to hepatitis.

(1) hepatitis does not affect potassium levels

(2) hepatitis does not affect sodium levels

(3) *correct*—deficiency of clotting factors can increase risk of hemorrhage

(4) hepatitis does not alter hemoglobin levels significantly

139. The nurse is caring for a client receiving total parenteral nutrition. Lab values are: glucose 72 mg/dL, chloride 98 mEq/L, sodium 138 mEq/L, potassium 3.0 mEq/L. Which of the following nursing actions is MOST appropriate?

1. Discontinue the TPN administration.
2. Notify the physician.
3. Administer IV glucose.
4. Check the client's vital signs.

Strategy: Answers are a mix of assessments and implementations. Does this situation require validation? No. Determine the outcome of the implementations.

(1) does not address the problem of hypokalemia; will cause hypoglycemia

(2) *correct*—normal plasma potassium level is 3.5–5.0 mEq/L; this client is low and needs replacement

(3) does not address the problem of hypokalemia

(4) situation does not require validation

140. The nurse is performing dietary teaching for a client with asymptomatic diverticular disease. The nurse knows that further teaching is required if the client makes which of the following statements?

1. "I'm glad that I can eat the tomatoes from my garden."
2. "I eat baby carrots as a snack almost every day."
3. "I mix several different kinds of lettuce for my evening salad."
4. "I only eat whole-wheat bread for my lunch sandwich."

Strategy: Determine the outcome of each statement. Is it desired?

(1) *correct*—contain indigestible roughage and seeds that may block the neck of a diverticulum

(2) encouraged for a high-fiber content to add bulk to stools

(3) encouraged for a high-fiber content to add bulk to stools

(4) encouraged to eat a diet high in cellulose and hemicellulose types of fiber, found in wheat bran and whole-wheat bread

141. The nurse is caring for a woman with pregnancy-induced hypertension (PIH) being treated with magnesium sulfate. The nurse would be MOST concerned if which of the following was observed?

1. Urine output decreased from 70 cc/h to 30 cc/h.
2. Respiratory rate increased from 14/min to 18/min.
3. Hypertonic patellar reflexes.
4. Blood pressure increased from 150/90 to 170/100.

Strategy: "MOST concerned" indicates a complication.
(1) *correct*—is metabolized and excreted by the kidneys; decrease in the urine output can lead to toxicity
(2) is a normal finding
(3) suggests magnesium deficiency
(4) suggests magnesium deficiency

142. A 12-year-old client is admitted to the pediatric unit in vaso-occlusive crisis from sickle cell anemia. As the nurse prepares the plan of care, which of the following orders should the nurse question?

1. Bedrest with bathroom privileges.
2. 2 liters oxygen via nasal cannula.
3. Maintain IV at keep open rate.
4. Administer analgesics as ordered.

Strategy: All answers are implementations. Determine the outcome of each answer choice. Is it desired?
(1) appropriate orders for this client
(2) appropriate orders for this client
(3) *correct*—adequate hydration must be maintained to prevent sickling and clumping of the affected cells
(4) appropriate orders for this client

143. A client on diazepam (Valium)for anxiety and nightmares and flashbacks about Vietnam. The nurse observes in this client: ataxia, confusion, dizziness, slurred speech. Which nursing actions are MOST appropriate?

1. Give the client a relaxation tape and send him to a quiet room.
2. Sit quietly with the client because he is currently having a flashback.
3. Recommend to the physician that the client be given medication to help him sleep.
4. Recommend that the physician evaluate the client's excessive use of the drug diazepam.

Strategy: The topic of the question is not clearly stated. Read answer choices for clues.
(1) does not deal with the physiologic problem
(2) inaccurate
(3) compound the problem because sleeping pills are cross-tolerant with diazepam
(4) *correct*—client is displaying symptoms of intoxication caused by excessive use of the drug diazepam, an indication of potential dependence

144. Which of the following indicates to the nurse a need for further teaching for a postoperative client using the incentive spirometer?

1. The client exhales with the spirometer in his mouth.
2. The client inhales with the spirometer in his mouth.
3. The client splints his incision before using the spirometer.
4. The client raises the head of his bed before using the spirometer.

Strategy: Answers are implementations. Determine the outcome of each answer choice. Is it desired?
(1) *correct*—incentive spirometry is designed to promote lung expansion by encouraging sustained maximal inspirations
(2) benefits the postoperative client during use of spirometry
(3) benefits the postoperative client during use of spirometry
(4) benefits the postoperative client during use of spirometry

145. During the health history, a teenaged girl states "I have no appetite and I've lost 4 pounds this week." It is MOST important for the nurse to take which of the following actions?

1. Notify the physician.
2. Weigh the client.
3. Continue with the interview.
4. Examine the abdomen.

Strategy: Answers are a mix of assessments and implementations. Does this situation require validation? Yes.

(1) passing the buck; no reason to contact the physician

(2) will be done as part of physical assessment; complete the interview

(3) *correct*—complete the health history, intervene before beginning physical assessment

(4) part of the physical assessment

146. The nurse observes a student nurse administer a Dulcolax suppository. Which of the following actions, if performed by the student nurse, would require an intervention by the nurse?

1. The client is instructed to hold his breath during insertion of the suppository.
2. The suppository is positioned to touch the wall of the patient's rectum.
3. The suppository is inserted 3–4 inches into the patient's rectum.
4. Lubricant is applied to the tip of the suppository before insertion.

Strategy: "Require an intervention" indicates an in *correct* action.

(1) *correct*—may cause rectal muscles to tighten, should breathe through mouth to relax

(2) acts by direct stimulation of mucosa, prevents suppository from being embedded in stool

(3) placement is *correct*

(4) lubricant eases insertion by preventing friction

147. The school nurse is interviewing a 15-year-old boy. The nurse would be MOST concerned if the adolescent made which of the following statements?

1. "I am so busy all the time that, at the end of the day, I am tired."
2. "Once in a while I fall over my feet when I am just walking around."
3. "I'm glad I don't get as sweaty as my friends when I work out."
4. "It is important that I wear clothes that are similar to what my friends wear."

Strategy: "MOST concerned" indicates something wrong.
(1) fatigue with increased activity is normal
(2) occasional awkwardness seen with growth spurts
(3) *correct*—should have increased in sweat production due to hormonal changes
(4) preoccupation with physical appearance normal.

148. The nurse is working in a pediatric clinic and takes a phone call from the mother of a three year-old who has vomited several times today. Which of the following instructions by the nurse is BEST?

1. "Offer your child some ice cream."
2. "Give your child some apple juice."
3. "Offer your child orange juice."
4. "Make some pudding for your child.'

Strategy: All answers are implementations. Determine the outcome of each answer choice. Is it desired?
(1) is part of a full liquid diet
(2) *correct*—clear liquids offered first; as child tolerates, then full liquids may be offered
(3) is part of a full liquid diet
(4) is part of a full liquid diet

149. A 32-year-old man with AIDS is admitted to the medical unit with complaints of fatigue, a persistent dry cough, and dyspnea on exertion. Vital signs are: BP 136/88, temperature 104°F (40°C), pulse 95, respirations 22. Which of the following actions by the nurse is BEST?

1. Administer a tepid sponge bath with the patient in a semi-Fowler's position.
2. Limit oral intake to a maximum of 2,000 cc of fluid per day.
3. Encourage the patient to perform passive ROM four times a day.
4. Suction the patient every 4 hours to maintain a patent airway.

Strategy: All answer choices are implementations. Determine the outcome of each answer choice. Is it desired?

(1) *correct*—reduces fever, provides comfort; bed elevated for respiratory distress
(2) needs fluids for hydration due to fever, encouraged to 3,000 cc/day
(3) activities paced to reduce shortness of breath and exhaustion; not best choice
(4) suctioning is performed PRN, unnecessary suctioning would irritate and increase secretions

150. Which of the following questions would BEST aid the nurse in assessing the orientation of a client on the psychiatric unit?

1. "Who is the president of the United States?"
2. "Do you remember my name?"
3. "What is your name?"
4. "What time is it?"

Strategy: Determine how each answer choice relates to orientation.
(1) some well-oriented people do not know the answer to this question, depending upon their age, educational level, etc.
(2) irrelevant
(3) *correct*—is a specific question related to orientation of person
(4) without consulting a watch or clock, most well-oriented people cannot answer this question

151. The nurse is performing teaching on a client with Bell's palsy. It is MOST important for the nurse to include which of the following instructions?

1. Use artificial tears 4 times per day.
2. Wear sunglasses at all times.
3. Avoid sudden movements of the head.
4. Change the pillowcase daily.

Strategy: Answers are all implementations. Determine the outcome of each answer choice. Is it desired?

(1) *correct*—paralysis of the eyelid allows the cornea to dry; patch can be used to keep the eyelid closed to prevent damage; drops and/or ointments are used to reduce chance of corneal damage

(2) no problem with intolerance to light

(3) is for clients with increased intraocular pressure

(4) Bell's palsy is not contagious

152. The nurse is reviewing client care documentation. Which of the following statements BEST indicates to the nurse that the staff requires additional instruction about documentation?

1. "Patient is very sad about the death of his daughter."
2. Patient states "I just can't get over my daughter's death."
3. "Patient frequently verbalizes about his daughter's death."
4. "Patient presents a sad face, stooped posture, and tear-streaked eyes."

Strategy: "Requires additional instruction" indicates in *correct* charting.

(1) *correct*—documentation is subjective

(2) quotes patient; *correct* documentation is complete and objective

(3) objective observation

(4) objective observation

153. The nurse finds a client unresponsive and making funny sounds. His arms and legs are stiff and jerking, and there is no verbal response. Which of the following actions should the nurse take FIRST?

1. Open the client's mouth and place a tongue blade between the teeth.
2. Position the client on his back, open the airway, and assess respiratory status.
3. Remain with the client and prevent him from injuring himself or falling out of bed.
4. Restrain the client's extremities and determine the neurological status.

Strategy: Answers are all implementations. Determine the outcome of each answer. Is it desired?

(1) may cause fracture

(2) impossible or inappropriate to carry out during a seizure

(3) *correct*—nurse should remain with client to prevent injury

(4) action is appropriate after a seizure

154. The nurse is monitoring a client with cholecystitis. The nurse would be MOST concerned if which of the following was observed?

1. Nausea.
2. Frequent belching.
3. Jaundice.
4. Right upper abdominal pain.

Strategy: "MOST concerned" indicates a complication.

(1) symptom of cholecystitis; does not necessarily indicate a complication

(2) symptom of cholecystitis; does not necessarily indicate a complication

(3) *correct*—jaundice indicates a possible stone in the bile duct, causing obstruction

(4) symptom of cholecystitis and does not necessarily indicate a complication

155. Which of the following statements by the client would indicate to the nurse that the client has an accurate understanding of the cause of her anxiety?

1. "When I get overly tired from working too hard, I begin to have severe headaches and nausea."
2. "I'm losing my mind. I can't think straight."
3. "My chest pounds and I can't catch my breath. I must be having a heart attack."
4. "Now that my mother has died, I've been thinking a lot about the way she abused me. I feel
very tense and sick."

Strategy: Think about what the words mean.
(1) indicates the client believes her anxiety is really exhaustion rather than stress
(2) common, but shows inaccurate client understanding of the source of the anxiety
(3) common, but shows inaccurate client understanding of the source of the anxiety
(4) *correct*—anxiety is often expressed as physical symptoms and can be triggered by situations in adult life that reawaken feelings of anger or anxiety unresolved from childhood

156. A 62-year-old man with peripheral vascular disease (PVD) states that he experiences leg pain frequently when walking, and asks the nurse in the clinic what he should do. The nurse should advise him to

1. lay down with his feet elevated above his heart when he experiences pain.
2. apply a heating pad to his legs for 15 minutes before walking.
3. walk until he experiences pain, then rest, and then resume walking.
4. do stretching exercises 20 minutes before starting to walk.

Strategy: All answers are implementations. Determine the outcome of each answer choice. Is it desired?
(1) decreases arterial flow to legs
(2) decreased sensitivity to pain may result in burns
(3) *correct*—exercise increases collateral circulation, should be encouraged
(4) stretching will not reduce pain due to intermittent claudication

157. Which of the following statements by an adult client indicates to the nurse a need for further teaching regarding care of a sigmoid colostomy?

1. "I hope to be able to go without a pouch soon."
2. "I'm irrigating my colostomy after each meal."
3. "My stoma is looking better all the time."
4. "It's not hard to change my pouch every several days."

Strategy: Determine the outcome of each answer choice. Is it desired?

(1) possible for many clients to go without a collection bag by performing routine irrigations

(2) *correct*—irrigation of sigmoid colostomy is not necessary more once a day and sometimesbevery two or three days, if at all

(3) normal reactions

(4) normal reactions

158. The nurse supervises a nurse's aide administer a soapsuds enema to a patient prior to abdominal surgery. Which of the following actions, if performed by the aide, would require an intervention by the nurse?

1. The aide holds the irrigation set 30 inches above the patient's rectum.
2. The aide inserts the irrigation tube 3 inches into the patient's rectum.
3. The aide positions the patient in Sims' position.
4. The aide warms the water to 105°F (40°C).

Strategy: "Require an intervention" indicates in *correct* behavior.

(1) *correct*—should be 12–18 inches; too high causes rapid distention and pressure in intestine causing rapid expulsion of solution, poor defecation, damage to mucous membranes

(2) should insert 3–4 inches

(3) placed descending colon at lowest point

(4) should be slightly higher than body temperature

159. The nurse is assessing a child with cystic fibrosis. The nurse would be MOST concerned if which of the following was observed?

1. The child is expectorating thick yellow mucus.
2. There is increased mucus production with postural drainage.
3. Exertional dyspnea increases during the day.
4. The child complains about difficulty breathing.

Strategy: Determine the significance of each answer choice and how it relates to cystic fibrosis.

(1) *correct*–is indicative of pneumonia
(2) increased mucous drainage is the purpose of postural drainage
(3) is not unusual for a child with cystic fibrosis
(4) is not unusual for a child with cystic fibrosis

160. The physician adds cholestyramine (Questran) 4 gm PO ac and hs to the medication regimen for a 66-year-old man. The client is also taking digoxin (Lanoxin) 0.125 mg PO qd and hydrochlorothiazide (Esidrix) 25 mg PO qd. The nurse assists the client to set up a medication schedule. Which of the following medication schedules is BEST?

1. 7 AM 8 AM 12 noon 5 PM HS Questran X X X X, Lanoxin X, Esidrex X
2. 7 AM 8 AM 12 noon 5 PM HS Questran X X X X, Lanoxin X, Esidrex X
3. 7 AM 8 AM 12 noon 5 PM HS
Questran X X X X Lanoxin X Esidrex X
4. 7 AM 8 AM 12 noon 5 PM HS Questran X X X X Lanoxin X Esidrex X

Strategy: Think about the action of each medication.

(1) Questran interferes with absorption of Digoxin and Esidrix
(2) Questran interferes with absorption of Digoxin and Esidrix; take Esidrix in early afternoon to prevent nocturia
(3) *correct*—Questran interferes with absorption of Digoxin
(4) Questran interferes with absorption of Digoxi

161. A 24-year-old woman comes to the prenatal clinic, pregnant for the first time. The client states she participates in a regular exercise program and asks the nurse if she should continue to do this during her pregnancy. Which of the following would be the BEST response by the nurse?

1. "You should limit your exercise because it may interfere with your ability to carry the child to term."
2. "You should restrict your exercise to taking brisk walks twice a day."
3. "You can exercise as much as you want, but you should cut back on your other activities."
4. "You can continue your regular exercise program, but you should rest when you are tired."

Strategy: "BEST" indicates there may be more than one response that you like. All answers are implementations. Determine the outcome of each answer choice. Is it desired?
(1) should limit strenuous exercise during last 4 weeks to decrease chance of low birth weight, still birth, or infant death
(2) should decrease weight-bearing exercises (running, jogging) and increase nonweightbearing exercise (swimming, stretching)
(3) should exercise no more than 3 times a week, would be too much to exercise as much as she wants
(4) **correct**—should exercise for 10–15 min, rest for 2–3 min, then exercise for 10 min, do stretching exercises to warm up before exercising

162. To best evaluate home compliance with metoclopramide (Reglan) for a three-month-old, the nurse should
1. observe the mother feeding the infant.
2. ask the mother about the infant's retention of feedings.
3. ask the mother how many wet diapers the baby has each day.
4. weigh the baby and compare to baseline weight.

Strategy: Topic of question is unstated. Read answer choices for clues.
(1) baby may have reflux after a home visit
(2) may reflect feeding retention; subjective information is not as reliable as objective measurements
(3) may reflect feeding retention; subjective information is not as reliable as objective measurements
(4) **correct**—is most accurate indicator of feeding retention

163. A staff member working in the newborn nursery complains to the nurse that even though s/he doesn't feel bad, s/he has been having loose stools for the last couple of days. Which of the following responses by the nurse is BEST?

1. "Make sure to wash your hands after going to the bathroom."
2. "Are you drinking plenty of fluids?"
3. "Describe to me how you are feeling."
4. "I'm going to reassign you to the orthopedics."

Strategy: Answers are a mix of assessments and implementations. Does this situation require validation?" No. Determine the outcome of each implementation.

(1) good hand washing is essential to preventing the spread of infection

(2) yes/no question; increase fluid to prevent fluid volume deficit

(3) staff member already stated that s/he feels OK

(4) *correct*—restrict from care of newborn, infants, or immunocompromised patients

164. The nurse is caring for a client in alcohol withdrawal. The nurse would expect the doctor to order which of the following oral medications to assist the client in decreasing the severity of the symptoms?

1. Amitriptyline (Elavil).
2. Trazodone (Desyrel).
3. Fluphenazine (Prolixin).
4. Chlordiazepoxide (Librium).

Strategy: Think about the action of each medication.

(1) antidepressant

(2) antidepressant

(3) antipsychotic medication

(4) *correct*—antianxiety medication is pharmacologically similar to alcohol; is used effectively as a substitute for alcohol in decreasing doses to comfortably and safely withdraw a client from alcohol dependence

165. Which of the following actions, if performed by the nurse, would be considered negligence?

1. Inserting a 16 Fr NG tube and aspirating 15 cc of gastric contents.
2. Administering Demerol IM to a patient prior to his using the incentive spirometer.
3. Administering ferrous sulfate (Feosol) 325 mg with coffee.
4. Initially administering blood at 5 cc per minute for 15 minutes.

Strategy: All answers are implementations. Determine the outcome of each answer choice. Is it desired?

(1) *correct* procedure; verify placement by checking pH of gastric aspirate

(2) reduces the pain, enables the patient to take a deep breath

(3) *correct*—do not give together, may impair iron absorption; give with orange juice

(4) *correct* procedure, start blood with normal saline and 19-gauge needle

166. A 26-year-old client was in a motor vehicle accident and has been admitted to an emergency room. Which of the following observations would indicate the need for the nurse to stay with the client?

1. Disorientation and irregular vital signs.
2. Irregular vital signs and hostility.
3. Rapid respirations and agitation.
4. Elevated vital signs and apprehension.

Strategy: Determine which situation is most unstable.

(1) *correct*—disoriented client with irregular vital signs represents a grave safety risk

(2) may increase the need for nursing interaction/assessment, but does not require the nurse to stay with client all the time

(3) may increase the need for nursing interaction/assessment, but does not require the nurse to stay with client all the time

(4) may increase the need for nursing interaction/assessment, but does not require the nurse to stay with client all the time

167. The nurse is assessing the emotional support available to a client who is starving herself. Which of the following questions would be MOST important for the nurse to ask in the assessment interview?

1. "What do you consider your ideal weight to be?"
2. "How does your eating pattern change when you are around other people?"
3. "What happens at home when you express opinions that are different from those of your parents?"
4. "What do you think about your present weight?"

Strategy: Think about what information is being asked for in each assessment question. Does it fit the situation?

(1) important question to ask during the assessment, but is not directly related to the issue of emotional support

(2) important question to ask during the assessment, but is not directly related to the issue of emotional support

(3) *correct*—is the question most likely to get at the ability of the parents to support the emotional needs of their children as separate human beings

(4) important question to ask during the assessment, but is not directly related to the issue of emotional support

168. The school nurse notes that one of the children has a copious watery discharge from the left eye, which is red. Which of the following actions, if taken by the nurse, is BEST?

1. Contact the child's parents to pick up the child.
2. Instruct the child to use a clean tissue each time he wipes his eye.
3. Contact the child's physician.
4. Obtain the child's temperature.

Strategy: Answers are a mix of assessments and implementations. Does this situation require validation? No. Determine the outcome of the interventions.

(1) *correct*—extreme tearing, redness, foreign body sensation are symptoms of viral conjunctivitis; highly contagious; children restricted from school until symptoms have resolved, 3–7 days

(2) appropriate action; more important to prevent child from spreading infection to other children

(3) passing the buck

(4) no reason to check temp, should remove child from environment

169. Nurse cares for child after hernia repair. Several hours after surgery, the nurse finds the knee gatch on the patient's bed elevated. The patient says he feels better with it elevated. The nurse should

1. check to see when the patient last received pain medication.
2. lower the knee gatch and place two pillows behind his knees.
3. check to make sure the knee gatch is not elevated more than 20°.
4. help the boy turn on his side and support his back with blankets.

Strategy: Answers are a mix of assessments and implementations. Does this situation require assessment? Yes.

(1) *correct*—patient indirectly indicates pain; assess before implementing action
(2) contraindicated, would compress blood vessels behind knee
(3) knee gatch used, compromise circulation, predispose to thrombus formation
(4) assessment should be done before implementation

170. A 22-year-old primipara is in active labor. As labor progresses, she becomes irritable and complains of feeling increasingly uncomfortable. The nurse notes she is 8 cm dilated. Which of these actions should the nurse take INITIALLY

1. Notify the physician of the patient's complaints.
2. Coach the patient in proper breathing and relaxation techniques.
3. Administer the standing order for meperidine (Demerol).
4. Reposition the fetal monitor to allow the patient to change positions.

Strategy: All answers are implementations. Determine the outcome of each answer. Is it desired?

(1) unnecessary, situation as described is normal
(2) *correct*—irritability and discomfort expected occurrences
(3) not first action; medications may depress infant's respirations after delivery; shouldn't give medication during transition
(4) situation as described is normal, not results of placement of fetal monitor

171. A 35-year-old man is receiving garamycin (Gentamycin) 500 mg q8h IV for a Pseudomonas infection in his leg. When the nurse walks into the patient's room. When he does not respond to the nurse's greeting, the nurse touches him on the shoulder. The patient jumps and acts startled. Which of the following actions, if performed by the nurse, is MOST important?

1. Ask the patient what he is thinking.
2. Monitor the color and sensation in the patient's leg.
3. Assess his temperature, pulse, and blood pressure.
4. Check the patient for tinnitus and hearing loss.

Strategy: "MOST important" indicates a priority question. All answers are assessments.

Determine why you would make each assessment and how it relates to the situation.

(1) assessment; does not address reason he was nonresponsive

(2) assessment; does not recognize that assessment needed because of the medication

(3) assessment; not relevant for issues raised in question

(4) *correct*—assessment; ototoxicity is serious adverse effect of aminoglycosides such as gentamycin

172. A 20-year-old woman comes to the outpatient clinic for complaints of vaginal itching. Which of the following recommendations, if given to the client by the nurse, is MOST appropriate?

1. "Supplement your diet with yogurt and dairy products."
2. "Douche with an over-the-counter preparation."
3. "Wash the area with soap and water several times a day."
4. "Wear underwear that is lined with a cotton crotch."

Strategy: All answer choices are implementations. Determine the outcome of each answer choice. Is it desired?

(1) contains bacilli that naturally exist in GI tract, no affect on vaginal pH

(2) may alleviate discomfort of vaginal discharge but would disrupt normal pH of vagina

(3) this frequency would cause dryness and increase itching in the area

(4) *correct*—more absorbent, allows for better circulation of air to body; dampness aggravates itching

173. A man has undergone a total laryngectomy due to carcinoma. The nurse is teaching the man and his wife how to suction the laryngectomy tube. Which of the following actions would indicate that teaching was effective?

1. The man selects a Yankauer tonsillar tip catheter to suction the laryngectomy tube.
2. The man takes several deep breaths before the suction catheter is inserted.
3. The man applies suction as he introduces the sterile catheter into the stoma.
4. The wife suctions the man's mouth and then the laryngectomy tube.

Strategy: "Teaching was effective" indicates a *correct* action.
(1) used for oral suctioning of mouth
(2) *correct*—hyperoxygenates and prevents anoxia
(3) apply suction only as catheter is withdrawn
(4) suction laryngectomy tube and then mouth

174. The parents of a newborn with a meningocele have been grieving the loss of their perfect child. After three days of grieving, the progress in their emotional status would be indicated to the nurse by which of the following comments?

1. "When will it be safe for us to hold our baby?"
2. "We would rather that you feed our baby."
3. "What did we do to cause this problem?"
4. "When do you anticipate our baby going home?"

Strategy: Determine what the words mean.
(1) *correct*—this comment indicates a desire to begin stroking and cuddling this baby; this
must happen before parents can provide physical care
(2) indicates a fear or a sense of insecurity with feedings
(3) indicates feelings of guilt
(4) is not specific to the question

175. Which statement, if made by the client with Cushing's syndrome, indicates to the nurse the need for further teaching?

1. "I realize I'll have to gradually begin an exercise program."
2. "I'm going to have to keep a close eye on my blood pressure."
3. "I'm not really worried about getting pneumonia this winter."
4. "I'll be eating foods low in carbohydrates and salt."

Strategy: "Need for further teaching" indicates an in *correct* response.
(1) exercise program should begin gradually
(2) client may develop hypertension related to sodium and water retention
(3) *correct*—statement indicates that the client does not realize there is an increased
susceptibility to infections
(4) diet should be low-carbohydrate, low-sodium, and high-protein

176. The nurse is caring for clients in a rehabilitation facility. To support the client to learn self-care, the nurse should take which of the following actions FIRST?

1. Provide instructions to complete an activity.
2. Observe client progress with an activity.
3. Establish the goal of the activity with the client.
4. Allow the client to complete as much self-care as desired.

Strategy: Remember the steps of the nursing process.
(1) appropriate; must first establish goal
(2) appropriate; but first establish goal
(3) *correct*—client commitment to completing or learning techniques for self-care is supported by participation in goal-setting
(4) appropriate; assess and plan before implementing

177. The nurse knows that which of the following information in a client's history would place her at greatest risk for suicide?

1. Two previous suicide attempts and increased use of alcohol.
2. Verbal threats without a specific plan.
3. Choice of a method that includes going to sleep and not waking up.
4. A specific plan but with ambivalence verbalized.

Strategy: Think about each answer and the relationship to suicide.
(1) *correct*—includes two factors that increase risk: the previous suicide attempt plus the
increase in alcohol use
(2) shows less risk because there is no specific plan
(3) includes a vague plan without a lethal method
(4) shows less risk because the client is ambivalent

178. The physician prescribes hydrochlorothiazide (Oretic) 50 mg PO daily for a client. The client also takes dexamethasone (Decaspray) 2 sprays in each nostril bid. The nurse should encourage the client to increase her intake of which of the following foods?

1. Chicken and low fat meats.
2. Dairy products and eggs.
3. Whole grain breads and fresh vegetables.
4. Citrus fruits and green leafy vegetables

Strategy: Determine what nutrients are being lost due to the medication. Determine which foods are highest in potassium.
(1) no need to increase protein
(2) no need to increase calcium intake
(3) no need to increase intake of roughage
(4) *correct*—need to increase intake of potassium-rich foods because of potassium loss from medications

179. The clinic nurse returns a phone call from a diabetic client who has been vomiting for 24 hours. It is MOST important for the nurse to instruct the client to

1. take only half of her regular insulin dose.
2. attempt to maintain her regular diabetic diet.
3. limit intake of sweets and sugar.
4. drink liquids as often as possible.

Strategy: All answers are implementations. Determine the outcome of each answer choice. Is it desired?

(1) diabetic should always take the regular dose of insulin, or alter it only according to serial glucose checks

(2) client is not tolerating PO foods

(3) sweets can be used as calories in this situation

(4) *correct*—diabetic ketoacidosis is frequently associated with dehydration; fluids should be encouraged

180. The nurse is caring for a patient admitted to the unit 3 days ago with second- and third-degree burns over 30% of her body. It would be MOST important for the nurse to report which of the following observations to the next shift?

1. CVP reading of 12 cm water pressure.
2. General muscle weakness and lethargy.
3. Heart rate of 100 beats per minute.
4. Systolic blood pressure of 105.

Strategy: Determine what each assessment is measuring and how it relates to burns.

(1) indicates adequate fluid resuscitation

(2) *correct*—muscle weakness and lethargy are signs of hypokalemia, which can occur on the third day after a burn; hypokalemia is caused by diuresis

(3) indicates adequate fluid resuscitation

(4) indicates adequate fluid resuscitation

181. An adult male client complains of hearing loss. While the nurse is irrigating his ear to remove cerumen for better observation of the tympanic membrane, the client comments that he is getting dizzy. The nurse would stop the procedure and

1. notify the physician immediately.
2. monitor for changes in intracranial pressure.
3. warm the irrigant and resume the procedure.
4. explore the canal with a cotton applicator.

Strategy: Answers are a mix of assessments and implementations. Are the assessments *correct*? No. Determine the outcome of the implementations.

(1) unnecessary

(2) assessment; client is not experiencing increased intracranial pressure

(3) *correct*—water that is too cool can elicit dizziness when it comes into contact with the tympanic membrane

(4) assessment; could compact the cerumen against the membrane; is never recommended

182. The nurse is caring for a patient 3 days after a spinal cord injury at the level of T-5. The patient complains of a pounding headache, and the nurse notes profuse sweating on the patient's forehead. Which of the following actions, if taken by the nurse, is BEST?

1. Determine the patency of the Foley catheter.
2. Place ice packs on the neck and head.
3. Elevate the head of the bed.
4. Apply a rigid cervical collar.

Strategy: Answers are a mix of assessments and implementations. Does this situation require assessment? Yes. Is the assessment appropriate? Yes.

(1) *correct*—autonomic dysreflexia may be precipitated by a full bladder; life-threatening complication characterized by severe hypertension; must be treated promptly to prevent a stroke

(2) client will need to be kept warm

(3) appropriate action; however, answer choice #1 is a higher priority

(4) does not address the immediate situation

183. After termination of preterm labor, the nurse confirms the ability of a client to monitor herself at home for fetal well-being if she can

1. count uterine contractions.
2. measure her urine output.
3. count fetal kicks.
4. weigh herself daily.

Strategy: Determine the significance of each assessment and how it relates to fetal well-being.

(1) might indicate the onset of premature labor
(2) relates to maternal well-being
(3) *correct*—ensures that the fetus is moving and makes the mother aware of the importance
of monitoring fetal movement daily
(4) relates to maternal well-being

184. The nurse is caring for patients on the pediatric unit. An eight-year-old patient with second- and third-degree burns on the right thigh is admitted. The nurse should assign the new patient with which of the following roommates?

1. A two-year-old with chickenpox.
2. A four-year-old with asthma.
3. A nine-year-old with acute diarrhea.
4. A ten-year-old with methicillin-resistant S. aureus (MRSA).

Strategy: Think about how the diseases are transmitted.

(1) infectious disease
(2) *correct*—patient not infectious; lowest risk of cross-contamination
(3) requires contact precautions; could cause infection in the burn patient
(4) could cause infection in the burn patient

185. The homecare nurse visits a client with a diagnosis of Addisons's disease. The nurse determines that teaching has been effective when the client makes which of the following statements?

1. "I'll take hydrocortisone (Cortef) in the morning."
2. "I'm glad that I will not have to change my dose of hydrocortisone (Cortef)."
3. "I'll increase my potassium by eating more bananas."
4. "This medicine probably won't affect my blood pressure."

Strategy: "Teaching has been effective" indicates a *correct* statement.

(1) *correct*—if steroids are taken at night, they may cause sleeplessness
(2) dosage has to be regulated according to the amount of stress
(3) client with Addison's disease has hyperkalemia
(4) steroids cause fluid retention, which can increase the blood pressure

186. The nurse is caring for a 23-year-old college student from China awaiting arthroscopic knee surgery. Which of the following observations would suggest that the client is anxious?

1. The client's skin is cool and dry.
2. The client shifts his position in bed frequently.
3. The client's pulse is 74, BP is 104/66.
4. The client answers questions appropriately.

Strategy: Determine how each answer relates to pain.

(1) would expect diaphoresis
(2) *correct*—nurse should assess for nonverbal cues such as increased restlessness, aggressive behaviors
(3) would expect increase in pulse and BP with anxiety
(4) does not indicate anxiety

187. The nurse is performing a home visit on a client with progressive multiple sclerosis (MS). The physician has just ordered cyclophosphamide (Cytoxan) and adrenocorticotropic hormone (ACTH). It is MOST important for the nurse to take which of the following actions initially?

1. Advise the client to purchase a wig or a hairpiece.
2. Instruct the client to decrease fluid intake.
3. Test the client's serum glucose concentration.
4. Observe for indications of gastrointestinal bleeding.

Strategy: Determine the outcome of each answer choice.

(1) *correct*—clients receiving cyclophosphamide usually develop alopecia four to five weeks after starting treatment

(2) should increase fluid intake to combat the side effect of hemorrhagic cystitis

(3) involves adverse effect of ACTH and should be monitored after treatment is initiated

(4) involves adverse effect of ACTH and should be monitored after treatment is initiated

188. A young Hispanic client who speaks little English is admitted to a medical-surgical unit with an increased temperature. Prior to performing a physical assessment, which of the following is the MOST appropriate nursing action?

1. Attempt to prepare the client with hand signals.
2. Show the client pictures of the physical exam process.
3. Contact an employee who speaks Spanish to translate.
4. Speak slowly to explain the physical assessment.

Strategy: Answers are implementations. Determine the outcome of each answer. Is it desired?

(1) less effective

(2) less effective

(3) *correct*—staff who speak other languages are usually noted by nursing administration for instances where a translator is the best option

(4) less effective

189. A client awakens during the night with dyspnea, severe anxiety, jugular vein distention (JVD), and frothy pink sputum. After the nurse begins oxygen at 4 L per nasal cannula, which of the following actions is MOST appropriate?

1. Place two pillows behind the head and elevate the legs.
2. Notify the physician about the change in the client's condition.
3. Increase IV fluids to liquefy the secretions.
4. Dim the lights and provide privacy.

Strategy: All answers are implementations. Determine the outcome of each answer choice. Is it desired?

(1) would increase fluids to the lungs

(2) *correct*—next priority is to notify the physician; signs indicate pulmonary edema

(3) would increase fluids to the lungs

(4) the nurse should stay with the client for reassurance

190. A 67-year-old man is returned to his room following a bronchoscopy. The client complains of thirst and requests ice chips. The physician has left an order for the patient to resume his regular diet. The nurse should

1. touch the back of the client's throat with a tongue depressor.

2. observe the client while he sucks on a few ice chips.

3. provide clear fluids to the client and advance to soft foods.

4. assess the client's tissue turgor and intake and output.

Strategy: Answers are a mix of assessments and implementations. Does this situation require assessment? Yes. Is there an appropriate assessment? Yes.

(1) *correct*—assessment, local anesthesia sprayed on throat, may interfere with swallowing

(2) assessment; need to check gag reflex first

(3) implementation; need to check gag reflex, may choke or aspirate

(4) assessment; does not address need to check gag reflex

191. A client at 38-weeks gestation is admitted in active labor. The nursing assessment reveals a decrease in the client's blood pressure to 90/50, and the fetal heart rate (FHR) is 130 and regular. Which of the following nursing actions would be MOST important?

1. Contact the physician.

2. Elevate the head of the bed.

3. Check the client's blood pressure and FHR every 30 minutes.

4. Place the client on her left side.

Strategy: Answers are a mix of assessments and implementations. Does this situation require validation? No. Determine the outcome of each implementation.

(4) *correct*—decrease in blood pressure is most likely due to pressure on the inferior vena cava, which occurs in the supine position (vena-caval syndrome); positioning client on her side will relieve pressure so that BP will increase

192. An elderly client is very confused and disoriented when he is admitted to the hospital from a long-term care facility. Which of the following would be a priority nursing assessment?

1. Determine his level of mobility when walking.
2. Evaluate his teeth and determine an appropriate diet.
3. Determine if a family member can remain at the bedside.
4. Assess the respiratory status and evaluate for hypoxia.

Strategy: Remember Maslow.
(1) not the highest priority
(2) not the highest priority
(3) not the highest priority
(4) *correct*—presence of hypoxia needs to be addressed immediately; hypoxia contributes to the confusion

193. The nurse is caring for a client who is scheduled for surgery. Immediately before transporting the client to the surgical area, the nurse should

1. check the client's vital signs.
2. check the client's identification bracelet.
3. ask the client to sign the operative permit.
4. administer the preoperative medications.

Strategy: Answers are a mix of assessments and implementations. Is the assessment appropriate? Yes.
(1) assessment; vital signs are checked prior to surgery, but not necessarily at the time the client is transferred
(2) *correct*—assessment; identity client must be completed before anything else
(3) implementation; must be done when the client is not rushed and has time to read and ask any questions regarding the permit before surgery is scheduled
(4) implementation; if the preoperative medication is not administered prior to this time, it will not achieve its maximum effectiveness

194. The initial nursing priority in working with a client diagnosed with dissociative disorder is to

1. assist the client to understand the relationship between anxiety and dissociation.
2. assess the client's level of and reason for memory loss.
3. assist the client to incorporate the dissociated material into conscious memories.
4. establish an honest, nonjudgmental, and safe relationship with the client.

Strategy: All answers are implementations. Determine the outcome of each answer choice. Is it desired?

(1) reasonable nursing goal that must be developed within a multidisciplinary approach in collaboration with the client after safe relationship is established

(2) reasonable nursing goal that must be developed within a multidisciplinary approach in collaboration with the client after safe relationship is established

(3) reasonable nursing goal that must be developed within a multidisciplinary approach in collaboration with the client after safe relationship is established

(4) *correct*—client is protecting him/herself from intense levels of anxiety that are beyond his/her coping abilities; client needs a safe, nonthreatening approach because s/he typically exhibits difficulty in establishing trusting relationships; if the client begins to feel "rushed," his/her anxiety level may rise, producing a potential for further dissociation

195. The nurse enters the room and discovers that the client has slurred speech, right-sided paralysis, and unequal pupils. Which of the following actions should the nurse take FIRST?

1. Call the physician.
2. Assess the respiratory status.
3. Determine the level of consciousness.
4. Perform a complete neurological evaluation.

Strategy: Answers are a mix of assessments and implementations. Does this situation require assessment? Yes. Is there an appropriate assessment? Yes.

(1) Physician will need to be notified after the nurse completes assessment of vital signs

(2) *correct*—assessing the respiratory status and ensuring the client has an open airway is the appropriate next step

(3) would need to be determined, but is not most appropriate next step

(4) would need to be done, but is not most appropriate next step

196. A 75-year-old woman undergoes a colonoscopy. During the post procedure period, it is MOST important for the nurse to monitor

1. the patient's ability to move her legs.
2. the patient's fluid and electrolyte balance.
3. the characteristics of the patient's stool.
4. the level of pain the patient experiences.

Strategy: Determine how each answer choice relates to a colonoscopy.

(1) spinal anesthesia not used
(2) *correct*—bowel prep and NPO status puts patient at high risk for imbalances
(3) will not have stools immediately after procedure due to bowel preparation
(4) not a painful procedure

197. A 54-year-old client with tertiary syphilis is admitted to a nursing unit. He is exhibiting signs of marked dementia and disorientation. Which of these actions should the nurse do INITIALLY?

1. Place the nurse call bell within reach.
2. Frequently observe the client's behavior.
3. Apply a vest-type restraint.
4. Provide an around-the-clock sitter.

Strategy: Answers are a mix of assessments and implementations. Does this situation require assessment? Yes.

(1) implementation; should not be assumed that the client will be able to use the call light appropriately
(2) *correct*—assessment; placing the client on frequent observation status would be the first action to ensure the client's safety
(3) implementation; should never be the first option exercised by a professional nurse; current standards require not only a physician's order but a time limit, the exact type of restraint to be used, and the specific rationale
(4) implementation; is not usually a nursing responsibility

198. Polyethylene glycolelectrolyte solution (GoLYTELY) is ordered for a client before a colonoscopy. The physician's office nurse explains to the client how to take the solution. Which of the following statements, if made by the client, indicates the need for further instruction?

1. "I need to drink 4 liters of the solution."
2. "If I drink it ice cold, it won't taste as bad."
3. "Once I finish drinking the solution, I can drink only water."
4. "I can use tap water to reconstitute the powder."

Strategy: "Need for further instruction" indicates you are looking for an in*correct* statement

(1) true statement
(2) *correct*—can cause hypothermia due to large quantity of solution ingested
(3) true statement
(4) true statement

199. In caring for a client with dementia, the nurse should give highest priority to which of the following goals?

1. Keeping the client alive.
2. Ensure that the client has an adequate fluid intake.
3. Returning the client to a functional role in the community.
4. Maintenance of an optimal level of functioning.

Strategy: Don't read into the question.

(1) would take priority if the client was experiencing delirium
(2) no information indicating intake is a problem.
(3) inappropriate because the client with dementia is not able to function at a higher level
(4) *correct*—dementia is characterized by severe, prolonged impairment, which is often irreversible, main focus of care is to keep client as healthy as possible for as long as possible

200. The nurse is caring for a patient after a craniotomy. The patient's history reveals breast cancer with metastatic lesions to the brain, and the patient has been receiving chemotherapy for one month. Postoperatively, the nurse would be MOST concerned if which of the following was observed?

1. Urine is foul-smelling and the urine specific gravity is 1.035.
2. The client's 24-hour fluid intake is 3,000 cc.
3. The client's 24-hour urinary output is 4,000 cc.
4. The client has diarrhea and excoriation of the anal area.

Strategy: Determine the significance of each answer choice and how it relates to a craniotomy.
(1) indicates either dehydration or infection
(2) intake is normal
(3) *correct*—indicates surgically induced diabetes insipidus; increased urine output with palecolored urine and low specific gravity
(4) is expected with a client in chemotherapy, but is not as high a priority as answer choice #3

201. The nurse is performing health screening at a shelter for the homeless. Which of the following nursing observations would most likely indicate the need for teaching about personal hygiene?

1. Fruity breath odor.
2. Foul-smelling stools.
3. Vaginal itching.
4. Red, swollen gums.

Strategy: Focus on the question.
(1) indicates the possibility of diabetic acidosis
(2) may be a result of poor fat absorption
(3) could be the result of antibiotic therapy and subsequent yeast infection
(4) *correct*—red, swollen gums can indicate pyorrhea, which is caused by improper cleaning and poor mouth hygiene

202. A 74-year-old woman is returned to the recovery room at the outpatient surgery center after cataract surgery. The nurse notes that the IV site in the client's left hand appears reddened and warm. Which of the following actions, if performed by the nurse, is BEST?

1. Call the physician to obtain an order to remove the IV cannula.
2. Apply cool compresses and continue to assess the IV insertion site.
3. Stop the IV infusion and remove the IV cannula.
4. Apply antibiotic ointment to the site and change the IV dressing.

Strategy: "BEST" indicates a priority question. All answers are implementations. Determine the outcome of each answer choice. Is it desired?
(1) if IV site is infected nurse can remove IV without an order
(2) should remove and replace IV in another site
(3) *correct*—if IV site is infected should be removed and restarted
(4) IV site should be changed if there are signs of infection

203. The nurse performs a diet history on a 35-year-old woman with AIDS hospitalized for a cytomegalovirus (CMV) infection of the gastrointestinal tract that has resulted in diarrhea. Which of the following food choices would indicate a need for the nurse to do further teaching?

1. A cup of beef bouillon, steamed white rice, and strawberry gelatin.
2. Clear chicken broth, two slices of white toast, and a serving of applesauce.
3. A cup of apple juice, cottage cheese, and three unsalted crackers.
4. Plain tea, a fresh fruit salad, and chocolate ice cream.

Strategy: "Further teaching is necessary" indicates an in *correct* response.
(1) low residue, contains protein
(2) low residue, high calorie
(3) low residue, contains protein
(4) *correct*—contain caffeine, roughage, dairy products

204. In coordinating community placement for an alcoholic schizophrenic client who has been homeless, the nurse should

1. collaborate with members of the client's family to explore placement options.
2. collaborate with the health care team and the client to schedule a predischarge visit to a residential placement facility.
3. visit the placement facility alone to make an independent decision about the facility, and report to the client and family.
4. review with the client specific rules of the facility.

Strategy: All answers are implementations. Determine the outcome of each answer choice. Is it desired?

(1) need to include client in decision-making

(2) *correct*—is important that multidisciplinary team discuss and collaborate with the client; needs support in decisions about discharge and residential living arrangements

(3) if the nurse visits independently of client sense of self-worth and decision-making

(4) reviewing rules with client prematurely can inhibit opportunity to explore feelings about this decision

205. The nurse is performing health screening at a senior citizen facility. A client states that she has been taking oral iron supplements for a month and complains of constipation. The nurse should adapt a diet plan to include

1. oatmeal, green beans, and celery.
2. strawberries and mushrooms.
3. grits, orange juice, and cheddar cheese.
4. pasta, buttermilk, and bananas.

Strategy: All answers are implementations. Determine the outcome of each answer choice. Is it desired?

(1) *correct*—contains foods highest in fiber (green vegetables and grains) to assist in counteracting constipation

(2) does not have as high a fiber content

(3) does not have as high a fiber content

(4) does not have as high a fiber content

206. Prior to discharging an infant home with his parents, which of the following statements, if made by the mother to the nurse, indicates a need for further teaching about newborn care?

1. "I will notify my physician about absence of breathing for 10 seconds."
2. "I will notify my physician about more than one episode of projectile vomiting."
3. "I will notify my physician if my baby's temperature is greater than 101°F."
4. "I will rock and cuddle my infant frequently to promote a sense of trust."

Strategy: "Need for further teaching" indicates that you are looking for an in *correct* **response.**

(1) *correct*—is normal for a neonate; apnea lasting longer than 15 seconds should be reported

(2) does not indicate a need for further teaching

(3) does not indicate a need for further teaching

(4) does not indicate a need for further teaching

207. A client recovering from streptococcal pneumonia has a chest x-ray that reveals a higher degree of atelectasis in the right lower lobe. Which of the following nursing interventions would be MOST appropriate?

1. Instruct the client to take deep breaths more frequently.
2. Reposition the client every hour to the right side.
3. Increase the frequency of incentive spirometry.
4. Change respiratory treatment to every 2 hours.

Strategy: All answers are implementations. Determine the outcome of each answer choice. Is it desired?

(1) would not be as effective as answer choice #3

(2) would actually decrease thoracic expansion of the chest wall on the right side

(3) *correct*—incentive spirometry is a quantifiable method to assess respiratory effort with deep-breathing exercises; increasing the frequency would be a sound nursing decision in an effort to improve the client's pulmonary status

(4) is not the best way to increase respiratory function.

208. While checking the patency of a Salem sump tube, the nurse finds stomach contents draining from the air vent. Which of the following nursing actions is MOST appropriate?

1. Insert water through the air vent.
2. Pull the sump tube back 2–3 inches.
3. Insert 30 cc air through the air vent.
4. Insert a new nasogastric tube.

Strategy: All answers are implementations. Determine the outcome of each answer choice. Is it desired?

(1) important not to put fluids through the air vent
(2) tube should not be withdrawn
(3) *correct*—clearing the air vent with air will reestablish proper suction in the Salem sump tube
(4) unnecessary

209. The home health nurse has been making home visits to follow the progress of a two-year-old boy with Tetralogy of Fallot. When the nurse visits the home, the child is found diaphoretic and short of breath. What should the nurse do FIRST?

1. Give the boy oxygen at 2 liters via nasal cannula.
2. Place the boy in the knee-chest or squatting position.
3. Administer morphine 0.1 mg/kg SQ to the boy.
4. Lay the boy in bed flat with his head elevated.

Strategy: All answers are implementations. Determine the outcome of each answer choice. Is it desired?

(1) not first intervention
(2) *correct*—knee-chest position treatment for cyanotic spells, enhances systemic venous return, dilates right ventricle, decreases the obstruction
(3) not done first
(4) should use knee-chest position

210. A four-month-old infant who had a temperature of 103°F (39.4°C) following his last DTP (diphtheria, tetanus, and pertussis) vaccine is seen in the clinic for another immunization administration. Prior to the nurse's administering the DTP, which of the following should be a priority?

1. Withhold the immunization.
2. Give half the dose in this injection.
3. Consult the physician about giving pediatric DT (diphtheria and tetanus).
4. Instruct the parents to give acetaminophen following administration of the full dose of DTP.

Strategy: Answers are implementations. Determine the outcome of each answer choice. Is it desired?
(1) withholding the diphtheria and tetanus vaccine is not indicated
(2) child would still receive the pertussis, which would probably cause another febrile reaction
(3) *correct*—fever over 103°F (39.4°C) in first 48 hours after DTP is a valid contraindication for pertussis vaccine
(4) would be *correct* if just the DT were given

211. A client has been taking levodopa (Larodopa) for tremors, shuffling gait, and rigidity. To evaluate the effectiveness of the medication, the nurse would document which of the following in the chart?

1. Client has had an increase in weight of 2 lb.
2. Client is less resistant to a respiratory infection.
3. Client has no tremors or shuffling gait.
4. Client is able to be more ambulatory.

Strategy: Determine how each answer choice relates to L-dopa.
(1) not result of the medication
(2) not result of the medication
(3) is unrealistic
(4) *correct*—is no cure for these symptoms, but levodopa (Larodopa) does reduce the rigidity and tremors, which facilitates mobility for the client

212. The homecare nurse makes a follow-up visit to a 38-year-old woman recently diagnosed with AIDS. Which of the following activities, if performed by the woman, indicates that the nurse's teaching has been effective?

1. The woman brushes her teeth once a day using a firm toothbrush.
2. The patient eats a large lunch at noon and a small dinner at 6 PM.
3. The patient changes the litter in her cat's litter box every day.
4. The patient takes docusate sodium (Colace) 300 mg once a day

Strategy: Think about what the words mean.

(1) should use a soft toothbrush 3 to 4 times/day to avoid injury to oral mucosa

(2) small frequent meals recommended to aid digestion

(3) AIDS patients shouldn't handle pet excreta

(4) *correct*—bowel programs, stool softeners, and laxatives reduce intestinal stasis and bacterial overgrowth

213. An alcoholic client who occasionally uses marijuana and cocaine is attending his second group therapy meeting. The client comments, "I am having difficulty sitting still. Am I bothering some of the group members? Maybe I should stop coming to these group meetings?" Which of the following nursing actions is MOST appropriate?

1. Encourage the client to share his problem with the group members.
2. Remove the client from the group and assess his needs.
3. Recognize that this is manipulative behavior and encourage the client to remain in the group.
4. Tell the client not to concern himself about the group members and to continue in the group.

Strategy: All answers are implementations. Determine the outcome of each answer choice. Is it desired?

(1) *correct*—client is experiencing some mild anxiety related to detoxification as well as participation in group process; needs reinforcement and encouragement to continue attending the group meetings and to share feelings

(2) is a result of anxiety

(3) is not manipulative behavior, but result of anxiety

(4) is a result of anxiety.

214. A 16-year-old boy is admitted to the hospital after sustaining a concussion due to an auto accident. The nurse would be MOST concerned if which of the following was observed?

1. The patient's blood pressure changes from 130/88 to 150/74.
2. The patient's pupils are equal and react to light and accommodation.
3. The patient has difficulty remembering what happened just before the accident.
4. The patient has a urinary output of 120 cc from 5 PM until 7 PM.

Strategy: "MOST concerned" indicates a complication.
(1) *correct*—increased systolic pressure and widening pulse pressure indicates increased intracranial pressure
(2) normal finding
(3) alteration in level of consciousness is symptom of cerebral edema but some amnesia for events immediately before accident is expected due to trauma
(4) 30 cc/hr normal finding

215. The public health nurse is caring for a child with impetigo. The nurse would be MOST concerned if which of the following was observed?

1. White patches on the buccal mucosa.
2. Hearing loss.
3. Respiratory wheezes.
4. Periorbital edema.

Strategy: "MOST concerned" indicates a complication.
(1) describes a fungal infection
(2) can be caused by many other factors
(3) can be caused by many other factors
(4) *correct*—indicative of poststreptococcal glomerulonephritis, a possible complication of
impetigo

216. The nurse overhears a conversation in the cafeteria between two nurses regarding a client's home situation. Which of the following actions is the MOST appropriate?

1. Report the incident to the nurse manager.
2. Join the conversation with the nurses.
3. Suggest that the nurses continue their conversation in private.
4. Ignore the incident since the nurse is not involved.

Strategy: Answers are implementations. Determine the outcome of each answer choice. Is it desired?

(1) may occur, but the situation requires immediate action that the manager may not be able to provide

(2) does not resolve the problem in a positive manner

(3) *correct*—client's confidentiality is being violated; it is nurse's responsibility to intervene to protect the client

(4) does not resolve the problem in a positive manner

217. Which of the following statements, if made by a 34-year-old man with Buerger's disease to the nurse, indicates that teaching has been effective?

1. "I should avoid taking analgesics if I become uncomfortable."
2. "The medication I am taking will prevent this disease from reoccurring."
3. "I should inspect my fingers and toes every day."
4. "It should keep track of how much fluid I drink during the day."

Strategy: Answers are a mix of assessments and implementations. Determine whether it is appropriate to assess or implement.

(1) feet cramps, claudication symptom of disease; pain control goal of treatment

(2) implementation; goal of medication is to prevent progression of disease

(3) *correct*—assessment; check for ulcer formation and gangrene; disease involves recurring inflammation of arteries and veins in upper and lower extremities, results in thrombus and occlusion, seen in men 20–35 years old; smoking is a causative factor; pain at rest and coldness major symptoms.

(4) assessment; fluids are not restricted or monitored

218. The nurse is performing a homecare visit on the family of a toddler. The nurse would be MOST concerned if which of the following was observed?

1. A bruise on the toddler's knee.
2. The toddler cries and is fearful when the parents leave.
3. The toddler's immunizations are not up-to-date.
4. The toddler throws a temper tantrum during an injection.

Strategy: Think about what the words mean?
(1) common assessment during the toddler years
(2) expected behavior for toddlers
(3) *correct*—most likely indicates a lack of concern for child's well-being and is a sign of poor quality of homecare
(4) expected behavior for toddlers

219. A female client has been taking levothyroxine sodium (Synthroid) 0.4 mg daily for four days. Which of the following findings should cause the nurse to recommend a change in the client's medication?

1. The client develops nervousness and difficulty sleeping.
2. The client states she has no energy and is "just tired."
3. The client has coarse hair and skin.
4. The client has a persistent weight gain.

Strategy: Think about each answer choice and how it relates to Synthroid.
(1) *correct*—suggest overdosage of thyroid hormone replacement therapy
(2) symptom of hypothyroidism, the reason for giving this medication
(3) symptom of hypothyroidism, the reason for giving this medication
(4) symptom of hypothyroidism, the reason for giving this medication

220. The nurse is preparing to insert a Foley catheter into a patient. It would be MOST important for the nurse to take which of the following actions?

1. Place all supplies close to the edge of the table.
2. Keep the field holding the supplies in front of the nurse.
3. Set up the field below the nurse's waist level.
4. Add only clean supplies to the field.

Strategy: All answers are implementations. Determine the outcome of each answer choice. Is it desired?

(1) would break sterile technique
(2) *correct*—represents the best technique for a sterile field
(3) would break sterile technique
(4) supplies should be sterile, would break sterile technique

221. A client with a severe thought disturbance has not been taking his medication and appears to be hallucinating more actively. The client claims that the medicine makes him drowsy during the day. Which of the following actions by the nurse is BEST?

1. Ask the physician to schedule the client's entire dose at bedtime.
2. Tell the client that he is getting sicker and must take his medicine.
3. Teach the client about the side effects of the medication.
4. Ask the family to talk to the client about this problem.

Strategy: Answers are implementations. Determine the outcome of each answer choice. Is it desired?

(1) *correct*—medication dose noncompliance is often associated with negative side effects and a multiple-dosing daily schedule; when client has only one daily dose at bedtime, is easier to remember to take medication; other advantage is that sedative effects of the drug peak while client is sleeping
(2) does not offer concrete solutions, encourage the client to act more childlike
(3) does not deal with the side effects of the medication
(4) passing the buck

222. A 56-year-old man is to receive peritoneal dialysis through a catheter inserted through a trocar. Which of the following nursing interventions is ESSENTIAL for the nurse to perform?

1. Maintain the client in a supine position during the procedure.
2. Weigh the client during the procedure and again 24 hours later.
3. Change the dwell time according to the client's tolerance during the procedure.
4. Check the client's BP and apical and radial pulses before the procedure.

Strategy: "ESSENTIAL" indicates a priority question. Answers are a mix of assessments and implementations. Is assessment required? Yes. What is the best assessment?

(1) implementation; on strict bedrest because of trocar but may be in semi-Fowler's position to prevent pressure of fluid on diaphragm

(2) assessment; should obtain weight, pulse, BP before procedure and again after

(3) implementation; dwell time is prescribed by physician

(4) *correct*—assessment; should obtain baseline vital signs

223. During a nonstress test (NST), the nurse observes several late decelerations. Which of the following nursing actions is MOST appropriate?

1. Reposition the client on her right side.
2. Notify the physician for further evaluation.
3. Document these results in the nurses notes.
4. Stop the oxytocin (Pitocin) immediately.

Strategy: Answers are implementations. Determine the outcome of each answer choice. Is it desired?

(1) does not resolve the immediate problem

(2) *correct*—appearance of any decelerations of the fetal heart rate (FHR) during NST should be immediately evaluated by the physician

(3) does not resolve the immediate problem

(4) in *correct* for this test; oxytocin (Pitocin) is not used for the nonstress test

224. A 60-year-old woman receives prochlorperazine maleate (Compazine) 10 mg IM before repair of a hernia under general anesthesia. The nurse would be MOST concerned if which of the following was observed six hours after surgery

1. An IV of 0.9% NaCl is infusing at 100 cc/hr.
2. The patient is sleepy but able to be aroused.
3. The patient has not voided since surgery.
4. There is a moderate amount of serosanguineous drainage on the abdominal dressing.

Strategy: "MOST concerned" indicates a complication.
(1) normal to replace fluids lost during surgery
(2) normal, due to general anesthesia
(3) *correct*—urine retention is side effect of medication and caused by general anesthesia
(4) some drainage expected

225. When doing an admission assessment on a client who has herpes zoster (shingles), it would be important for the nurse to determine which of the following?

1. When the client developed this allergic reaction and how long it has lasted.
2. If the client has eaten any new foods within the past 24 hours.
3. If the client has a history of fever blisters or canker sores.
4. If the client comes in contact with anyone with chicken pox.

Strategy: Determine how each assessment relates to herpes zoster.
(1) herpes zoster is caused by a virus; it is not an allergic reaction
(2) herpes zoster is not caused by a food allergy
(3) herpes simplex is related to fever blisters and cancer sores, not herpes zoster
(4) *correct*—close relationship between the virus that causes herpes zoster (shingles) and chicken pox virus

226. A client is admitted to the emergency room with complaints of crushing chest pain, shortness of breath, and left arm pain. Which of the following actions, if taken by the nurse, is BEST?

1. Administer oxygen.
2. Place in a semi-Fowler's position.
3. Administer morphine sulfate.
4. Administer lidocaine.

Strategy: All answers are implementations. Determine the outcome of each answer choice. Is it desired?

(1) would be implemented after answer choice #3 was implemented

(2) the position should be high Fowler's

(3) *correct*—the priority is to decrease the pain; this will decrease the metabolic needs, which will result in a decrease in the cardiac demands; morphine reduces preload and afterload pressures, increasing cardiac output

(4) there is no indication of ventricular tachycardia

227. The nurse is conducting a class on the changes associated with aging at a senior citizen center. The nurse would be MOST concerned if a client made which of the following statements?

1. "I seem to get colds more often now than I did years ago."
2. "I'm about an inch shorter now than I was when I was working."
3. "I don't mind cooking, but eating doesn't appeal to me much anymore."
4. "I've been sleeping with fewer blankets over me lately."

Strategy: "MOST concerned" indicates that you are looking for something wrong. Think about the answer choices and how each relates to aging.

(1) normal change associated with aging process

(2) normal change associated with aging process;due to collapse of vertebral column

(3) normal change associated with aging process; may be due to depression

(4) *correct*—usually becomes intolerant to cold

228. An elderly client has had a subtotal gastrectomy. The client has received meperidine (Demerol) 75 mg and hydroxyzine hydrochloride (Vistaril) 50 mg IM. The nurse is MOST concerned if which of the following was observed?

1. Tachypnea.
2. Lethargy.
3. Hypertension.
4. Disorientation.

Strategy: Think about each answer choice and how it relates to the medication.
(1) inaccurate
(2) expected finding
(3) inaccurate
(4) *correct*—elderly are prone to paradoxical reactions and can become agitated and disoriented

229. A six-year-old girl is admitted to the pediatric unit with a diagnosis of bacterial meningitis. As the nurse explains care to the parents, they ask how long their daughter will need to be in a room by herself. Which response by the nurse would be MOST appropriate?

1. "It depends on the results of her blood counts."
2. "Patients like her are usually in isolation a couple of days or so."
3. "Isolation can usually be stopped 24 hours after the start of antibiotic therapy."
4. "When she has been afebrile for 48 hours, we will move her."

Strategy: "MOST appropriate" indicates that two answer choices will be similar.
(1) not accurate; may depend on negative lumbar puncture
(2) nontherapeutic, dismissive tone
(3) *correct*—treated with penicillin; IV fluids, isolation for 24 h after the start of antibiotic therapy to prevent respiratory transmission
(4) inaccurate; don't use medical terms without explanation

230. The nurse is caring for a client with a three-chamber water-seal drainage system (Pleur-evac). While assisting the man from the bed to the chair, the drainage tubing becomes disconnected from the Pleur-evac. The nurse should

1. insert the tubing in a container of sterile saline solution.
2. cut the tubing two inches from the end and clamp securely.
3. reconnect the tubing to the Pleur-evac container.
4. connect the tubing to a new Pleur-evac container.

Strategy: All answers are implementations. Determine the outcome of each answer choice. Is it desired?
(1) *correct*—prevents air from reentering the pleural space
(2) clamping tube alters the pressure in the pleural space
(3) must maintain sterility of equipment
(4) need to do something while additional equipment is obtained

231. Several hours after an oxytocin (Pitocin) infusion is started, the client's contractions are sustained over two minutes. Which of these nursing actions would be MOST important?

1. Discontinue the IV Pitocin.
2. Administer oxygen.
3. Reposition the client.
4. Decrease the IV Pitocin rate.

Strategy: All answers are implementations. Determine the outcome of each answer choice. Is it desired?
(1) *correct*—sustained contractions can lead to a ruptured uterus and/or fetal distress
(2) important if fetal distress is apparent
(3) important if fetal distress is apparent
(4) not appropriate for situation; client would continue to receive Pitocin

232. The nurse is teaching a client how to understand and deal with his hallucinations. Which of the following indicates to the nurse that teaching has been successful?

1. The client reports that he is feeling anxious and requests his radio and headphones in
anticipation of "the voices."
2. The client sleeps during the day and avoids going to his assigned activities.
3. The client requests PRN medication between the two regularly scheduled doses.
4. The client reports that he is angry and wishes to leave the hospital immediately.

Strategy: All answers are implementations. Determine the outcome of each answer choice. Is it desired?
(1) *correct*—client is connecting his voices with feeling of anxiety and is taking action to get rid of the voices
(2) gives no indication of learning a positive behavior
(3) does not indicate any level of understanding of the cause of the symptoms
(4) does not indicate any level of understanding of the cause of the symptoms

233. The nurse prepares a 67-year-old man for an intravenous pyelogram (IVP). Which of the following statements, if made by the client to the nurse, would indicate that teaching has been effective?

1. "I may feel a fluttery sensation when the catheter is inserted."
2. "The test may cause spasms and shooting pains in my back."
3. "I may experienced a hot feeling and my skin may become flushed."
4. "I may become lightheaded and have a desire to cough."

Strategy: "Teaching has been effective" indicates you are looking for a *correct* response.
(1) these symptoms experienced during cardiac catheterization as catheter is passed into left ventricle, not seen with IVP
(2) does not occur during IVP
(3) *correct*—may be accompanied by nausea caused by dye injection
(4) not associated with IVP

234. The nurse is caring for a patient one day after a thoracotomy. The patient is receiving 40% humidified oxygen. Arterial blood gas (ABG) results are: PaO2 90 mm Hg, PaCO2 49 mm Hg, pH 7.30, HCO3 26 mEq/L. Which of the following nursing actions is BEST?

1. Position in high Fowler's and encourage coughing and deep breathing; evaluate airway patency.
2. Place in prone position and request respiratory therapy to perform postural drainage and percussion therapy.
3. Call the physician to advise about the arterial blood gas report; anticipate increase in oxygen percentage.
4. Administer antianxiety agent and assist the patient with a rebreathing device to increase oxygen levels.

Strategy: All answers are implementations. Determine the outcome of each answer choice. Is it desired?
(1) *correct*—client is experiencing respiratory acidosis from decreased ventilation; increasing quality of ventilation by removing secretions may resolve the problem
(2) is used for chronic airway problems
(3) oxygen levels are within normal range; need to take action to improve ventilation before notifying the physician
(4) treatment for respiratory alkalosis

235. A 20-year-old, gravida 1, para 0 woman comes to the clinic for her first routine prenatal exam. During the physical assessment, the client informs the nurse that she is unsure of the date of her last menstrual period. Which of the following assessments would best assist the nurse in determining her expected date of confinement (EDC)?

1. The presence of Hegar's sign.
2. A positive pregnancy test.
3. The presence of quickening.
4. Auscultation of the fetal heartbeat.

(1) probable sign of pregnancy

(2) probable sign of pregnancy

(3) presumptive sign of pregnancy

(4) *correct*—fetal heartbeat can be heard at 12 weeks; is a positive sign of pregnancy

236. A 40-year-old man is hospitalized with a fractured pelvis following an automobile accident. A female nurse is administering routine morning care when the patient tells the nurse that he finds her extremely attractive and would like her to come back to visit him that evening after work. Which of the following responses by the nurse would be BEST?

1. "I appreciate the compliment you paid me, but why did you ask me that?"

2. "That kind of interaction is not appropriate.Why don't you finish shaving?"

3. "It is interesting that you feel that way. Do I remind you of someone?"

4. "You seem to be attracted to me, but I don't feel the same way."

Strategy: Remember therapeutic communication.

(1) minimizes comment and asks "why" which is nontherapeutic

(2) *correct*—uses technique of acknowledging and redirecting

(3) observing and clarifying not appropriate in this situation

(4) reflecting and rejection not appropriate in this situation

237. Four days ago the physician prescribed lithium carbonate (Lithobid) 600 mg TID for a 52-yearold man. He returns with his wife to the outpatient clinic for evaluation. What teaching regarding the medication is MOST important for the nurse to reinforce with the man and his wife?

1. He should check for ankle swelling and decreased urinary output.

2. Keep a log of the time of day he takes his medication and how he is feeling.

3. He should call the clinic if he develops tremors, muscular weakness, or ataxia.

4. Because of the medication, he should be experiencing remission of his symptoms.

Strategy: Determine how each answer relates to lithium.

(1) should check for ankle edema, lithium causes polyuria (increase in urinary output) and dehydration

(2) should check weight daily and have lithium levels checked 8–12 h after first dose, 2–3 times a week the first month, then weekly to monthly while on maintenance

(3) *correct*—50% will develop dose-related tremors, signs of toxicity are diarrhea, vomiting, drowsiness, muscular weakness, ataxia

(4) takes 1–2 weeks before patient will see results

238. The nurse is caring for an eight-year-old child after a tonsillectomy. The nurse would be MOST concerned if which of the following was observed?

1. Heart rate of 88 beats per minute.
2. Expectorating bright red secretions.
3. 30 ml of dark brown secretions.
4. Infrequent swallowing.

Strategy: Determine the significance of each answer choice and how it relates to a tonsillectomy.

(1) normal rate for an 8-year-old

(2) *correct*—secretions that are bright red indicate hemorrhage

(3) would be expected because of the surgical procedure

(4) would be expected after the surgery because of discomfort

239. A client recently admitted to labor and delivery states that she is having severe discomfort with contractions. The nursing assessment reveals that the client is 3 cm dilated. The nurse assists the client through guided imagery. Ten minutes later the client is more agitated. The nurse should

1. reteach the exercise.
2. reposition the client.
3. turn on the television.
4. ambulate the client.

Strategy: All answers are implementations. Determine the outcome of each answer choice. Is it desired?

(1) increase in discomfort and agitation indicates that pain management through guided imagery is not successful

(2) *correct*—increase in discomfort and agitation indicates that pain management through guided imagery is not successful, so it should be discontinued and another nursing intervention implemented, such as repositioning the client

(3) might distract the client, but would not be as effective as answer choice #2

(4) would increase the pain

240. The nurse is caring for a client in hypovolemic shock. Which of the following would indicate a therapeutic response to volume replacement?

1. Urine output increased to 40 cc per hour.

2. Blood glucose of 180 mg/dL, serum potassium of 4.0 mEq/L.

3. CVP of 5 cm water, pupils equal and reactive.

4. Pulse rate of 110 with no dysrhythmias.

Strategy: Think about how each answer choice relates to adequate fluid volume.

(1) *correct*—primary objective of fluid replacement is to perfuse vital organs; increase in urine output to a normal range indicates that kidneys are adequately perfused; other major organs are being perfused also

(2) does not give any indication of adequate fluid replacement

(3) CVP of 5 cm water is in the low range,does not indicate adequate tissue perfusion

(4) client is tachycardiac; absence of arrhythmias does not indicate tissue perfusion

241. The nurse is preparing to examine the client's thyroid gland. Which of the following statements, if made by the nurse, is BEST?

1. "Would you like a band-aid?"

2. "Here is a glass of water."

3. "I will be using this tape measure."

4. "Please use this specimen cup."

(1) not an invasive procedure

(2) *correct*—drinking water facilitates swallowing during examination of thyroid

(3) don't measure with a tape measure

(4) no specimen is obtained

242. Which nursing action is MOST appropriate when an infant is admitted for fever, poor feeding, irritability, and a bulging fontanelle?

1. Perform neurological checks every four hours.
2. Place the client on droplet precautions.
3. Monitor the client's urine output closely.
4. Encourage fluid intake.

(1) assessment; not a priority

(2) *correct*—implementation; classic signs of meningitis; client should be isolated from other clients

(3) assessment; not a priority

(4) implementation; inappropriate for this situation

243. The physician orders an analgesic to be administered to a woman in labor who is nine cm dilated and having contractions every three minutes, lasting for 50 seconds. Which of the following nursing actions is MOST important?

1. Identify the client prior to administering medication.
2. Calculate the amount of medicine to be administered.
3. Hold the medication and document the order in nursing notes.
4. Notify the physician regarding the status of the contractions.

Strategy: Answers are implementations. Determine the outcome of each answer choice. Is it desired?

(1) client should not receive analgesic

(2) not appropriate for this situation

(3) does not address the immediate problem

(4) *correct*—information indicates that woman is in transition phase; analgesics should not be administered during transition phase

244. The nurse questions the family of a patient admitted with hyperglycemic hyperosmolar nonketotic syndrome (HHNK). The nurse should expect which of the following information to be contained in the patient's history?

1. The patient was diagnosed with type I diabetes mellitus (IDDM) four years ago.

2. The patient has a history of 3+ ketones in his urine.

3. The patient is 20 lb overweight and smokes a pack of cigarettes a day.

4. The patient is 66 years old and takes propranolol (Inderal) 20 mg PO tid.

Strategy: Think about the cause of each answer choice and how it relates to the situation.

(1) usually seen with type II diabetes (NIDDM)

(2) ketosis usually not seen with this condition

(3) no relationship to weight or smoking

(4) *correct*—seen after 50 years old, age-related changes in thirst perception results in dehydration and decrease in urine-concentrating abilities of the kidney

245. During a well-baby check-up the nurse evaluates the reflexes of a six-month-old child. The nurse would be MOST concerned if which of the following was observed?

1. Presence of a positive Babinski reflex.

2. Extrusion reflex when feeding.

3. Able to grasp objects voluntarily.

4. Rolls from abdomen to back at will.

Strategy: "MOST concerned" indicates you are looking for a complication.

(1) disappears at approximately one year

(2) *correct*—extrusion reflex disappears between three and four months of age

(3) normal occurrence at this age level

(4) normal occurrence at this age level

246. The nurse is reviewing the record for a patient with a chest tube attached to a Pleur-evac system. The nurse evaluates that which of the following nursing actions was appropriate?

1. "Chest tube was clamped."
2. "Pleur-evac next to bed."
3. "Suction decreased to 15 cm."
4. "Chest tube disconnected from the Pleur-evac."

Strategy: All answers are implementations. Determine the outcome of each answer choice. Is it desired?

(1) chest tube should not be clamped

(2) *correct*—Pleur-evac should be maintained below the level of the chest to prevent back flow of fluid and air into the pleural space

(3) there is no reason to decrease the level of suction

(4) do not disconnect a chest tube

247. The nurse is performing teaching on a client that is being discharged on dexamethasone (Decadron) 0.75 mg PO qd. The nurse knows that teaching has been successful if the client makes which of the following statements?

1. "I will take my medication with orange juice in the morning."
2. "I will take my medication with dinner."
3. "I will take my medication three hours after eating."
4. "I will take my mediation before I eat breakfast."

Strategy: "Teaching was successful" indicates a *correct* response.

(1) contains in *correct* information about the administration of steroids

(2) *correct*—oral steroids have ulcerogenic properties and need to be administered with meals

(3) contains in *correct* information about steroid administration

(4) contains in *correct* information about steroid administration

248. Four days after a client has an abdominal perineal resection, which of the following signs is MOST important for the nurse to report to the physician?

1. Moderate amount of serosanguineous drainage on the abdominal dressing.
2. Nausea, vomiting, and increased abdominal distention.
3. Moderate amount of yellow-green nasogastric drainage and decreased urine output.
4. Urinary output via Foley catheter 120 cc over a four-hour period.

Strategy: Determine how each answer choice relates to a complication after surgery.

(1) expected after this type of surgery

(2) *correct*—symptoms indicate paralytic ileus and should be reported to the physician

(3) nasogastric drainage is expected after this type of surgery, but amount of urinary output is not expected to change significantly

(4) normal output via Foley

249. A 75-year-old man with Alzheimer's disease frequently wanders down the halls of the extended care facility and displays restless agitation. The physician orders a vest restraint. When the nurse takes the restraint to the room, the patient refuses to put it on. It is MOST important for the nurse to

1. take the restraint away and check the patient frequently.
2. notify the physician immediately that the patient refused the restraint.
3. have a coworker hold the patient and gently apply the restraint.
4. exchange the vest restraint for wrist restraints.

Strategy: "MOST important" indicates a priority question. All answers are implementations. Determine the outcome of each answer choice. Is it desired?

(1) *correct*—as long as behavior is not unsafe, nurse should try other methods to engage patient in activities to reduce wandering

(2) not first or most important action of nurse, patient is primary responsibility

(3) should not forcibly restrain patient

(4) will make agitation worse, shouldn't restrain patients against their will

250. A client with urinary frequency, burning, and a temperature of 102°F (38.8°C) is instructed by the nurse to collect a urine specimen for culture and sensitivity. The nurse knows that teaching has been successful if the client makes which of the following statements?

1. "I will call the lab before I collect my urine."

2. "I will drink several glasses of water before I collect my urine."

3. "I will collect the specimen using aseptic technique."

4. "I will discard my first voiding in the morning."

Strategy: All answers are implementations. Determine the outcome of each answer choice. Is it desired?

(1) unnecessary for the collection

(2) unnecessary for the collection

(3) *correct*—aseptic technique decreases contamination with organisms

(4) unnecessary for the collection

251. The nurse is caring for clients in the same day surgery unit. It is MOST important for the nurse to further investigate which of the following client statements?

1. "I take an herbal dietary supplement to lose weight."

2. "I had acute glomerulonephritis ten years ago."

3. "I perform yoga and walk on my treadmill everyday."

4. "I took my blood pressure medication three hours ago."

Strategy: Determine the significance of each statement and how it relates to surgery.

(1) *correct*—some appetite suppressants resemble amphetamines and may cause palpitation and hypertension; notify the physician

(2) nephritis usually caused by beta-hemolytic strep elsewhere in the body; not priority

(3) good health habits

(4) medication for cardiac disease and hypertension may be taken at least two hours before surgery with small sips of water

252. A client with sudden onset of deep vein thrombosis (DVT) is started on an IV heparin drip. Which of the following orders should the nurse question?

1. Warm moist packs to the affected leg.

2. Elevate the foot of the bed six inches.

3. Commode privileges without weight bearing.

4. Elastic stockings on unaffected leg.

Strategy: "Question orders" indicates an in *correct* order.

(1) *correct*—warm moist heat is used to relieve the pain and treat the inflammation

(2) appropriate therapy

(3) appropriate therapy

(4) appropriate therapy

253. The nurse knows that which of the following diversional activities is most appropriate for a tenyear- old female client recovering from a sickle-cell crisis?

1. Walking in the hall 20 minutes twice a day.

2. Watching the cartoon channel all day.

3. Collecting pictures of favorite stars from magazines.

4. Putting together large-pieced wooden puzzles.

Strategy: All answers are implementations. Determine the outcome of each answer choice. Is it desired?

(1) will not conserve her much-needed energy

(2) an isolating activity

(3) *correct*—collecting is an activity that is important to school-aged children

(4) appropriate for preschool-aged children

254. The nurse cares for a client after a thyroidectomy. The nurse would be MOST concerned if which of the following was observed?

1. Tension and muscle spasm of the hand when a blood pressure cuff is applied to the arm and inflated.
2. Absence of facial movement when the muscles of the facial nerve or branches of the nerve are tapped.
3. Pain in the neck when pulling self to a sitting position or with sudden head movements.
4. Blood pressure readings that remain 10 points below the preoperative readings.

Strategy: "MOST concerned" indicates a complication.
(1) *correct*—positive Trousseau's sign, indicates tetany, surgery may damage parathyroid glands and cause a decrease in serum calcium
(2) negative Chvostek's sign, positive sign indicates low serum calcium
(3) expected after surgery in neck area
(4) expected; may be caused by blood loss during surgery

255. The nurse is caring for a client with radium implant. It is MOST important for the nurse to take which of the following actions?

1. Evaluate the position of the applicator every two hours.
2. Place the client on a low-residue diet to decrease bowel movements.
3. Encourage the use of the bedside commode every one to two hours.
4. Decrease fluid intake to decrease radiation in the bladder.

Strategy: Answers are a mix of assessments and implementations. Is the assessment appropriate? No. Determine the outcome of each implementation.
(1) assessment, should be checked every eight hours
(2) *correct*—implementation; bowel movements can dislodge radium implant; this diet will decrease amount of stool and number of bowel movements
(3) implementation; client is on strict bedrest
(4) implementation; decreasing fluids will not alter exposure to radiation; client should have a high fluid intake

256. The nurse is supervising a student nurse administer a tube feeding to a client with a tracheostomy. The nurse would intervene if which of the following was observed?

1. The student nurse places the client in a supine position.
2. The student nurse aspirates and returns the residual stomach contents.
3. The student nurse checks the pH of the gastric content.
4. The student nurse checks the bowel sounds for 5 minutes in each quadrant

Strategy: Determine the outcome of each answer choice.
(1) *correct*—to minimize the risk for aspirations, the client should be maintained in semi- Fowler's position
(2) appropriate intervention
(3) appropriate intervention
(4) appropriate intervention

257. During the first trimester of pregnancy, a client experiences hyperemesis, which results in a decrease in weight, poor skin turgor, and a chloride deficiency. Which of the following nursing orders should the nurse implement FIRST?

1. Offer fluids every hour as tolerated.
2. Complete an intake and output record every four hours.
3. Start an IV immediately upon admission.
4. Perform a daily weight every morning.

Strategy: Answers are a mix of assessments and implementations. Is the assessment appropriate? No. Determine the outcome of the implementations.
(1) *correct*—offering fluids at frequent intervals will increase hydration status
(2) contains a plan to evaluate the status of hydration
(3) contains a plan formulated from the physician's orders; the question refers to nursing orders
(4) assessment; is an appropriate action for evaluating the client, but it does not meet hydration needs

258. The nurse is supervising a nurse's aide transfer of a 58-year-old woman from the bed to the chair after a right total hip replacement. The nurse should intervene if which of the following was observed?

1. The nurse's aide helps the woman to a sitting position.
2. The nurse's aide positions the chair at a 90° angle to the bed.
3. The nurse's aide stands on the same side of the bed as the patient's unaffected side.
4. The nurse's aide pivots the patient on the unaffected leg.

Strategy: "Nurse should intervene" indicates an in *correct* action.
(1) helps prevent orthostatic hypotension and dizziness
(2) right way to place chair
(3) *correct*—should stand on affected side
(4) right way to move patients

259. A client is scheduled for a myelogram because of complaints of severe lumbar pain. Which of the following nursing interventions would be MOST important for this procedure?

1. Inform the client about being NPO prior to the test.
2. Encourage ambulation after the test.
3. Encourage fluids prior to and after the test.
4. Instruct the client to remain prone for 24 hours.

Strategy: All answers are implementations. Determine the outcome of each answer choice. Is it desired?
(1) will be NPO for 4 to 6 hours, but not most important
(2) bedrest may be maintained for as long as 24 hours
(3) *correct*—fluids promote excretion of the dye and also facilitate formation of spinal fluid
(4) should have the head elevated at 30° for 24 hours

260. **A woman states she is in the 39th week of gestation with her second baby and has been having contractions for several hours. The woman has been unable to obtain assistance because the roads are impassable. The nurse assists with the delivery of the infant. Once the head is delivered, it is MOST important for the nurse to**

1. instruct the woman to bear down and push.
2. turn the infant's head in a clockwise direction.
3. check the infant's neck for the umbilical cord.
4. ask the woman to pant through her mouth.

Strategy: Answers are a mix of assessments and implementations. Does this situation require assessment? Yes. Is there an appropriate assessment? Yes.

(1) implementation; should bear down with contractions, but not most important

(2) implementation; head will rotate without assistance to right or left, should not be turned

(3) *correct*—assessment; infant could become anoxic if cord is around neck

(4) implementation; should bear down with contractions

261. **The nurse is caring for a client with a bleeding duodenal ulcer. The nurse would be MOST concerned if the patient reported taking which of the following medications?**

1. Ranitidine hydrochloride (Zantac) 150 mg PO.
2. Metoclopramide hydrochloride (Reglan) 15 mg PO.
3. Sucralfate (Carafate) 1 gm PO.
4. Famotidine (Pepcid) 20 mg PO.

Strategy: Think about the action of each medication.

(1) inhibits action of histamine at receptor site of parietal cells decreasing gastric acid secretion, used for short-term treatment of duodenal and gastric ulcers

(2) *correct*—stimulates motility of upper GI tract, contraindicated with possible hemorrhage of GI tract, used to treat nausea of chemotherapy

(3) adheres to and protects ulcer surface by forming a barrier, used for short-term treatment of duodenal ulcer

(4) inhibits action of histamine at receptor site of parietal cells decreasing gastric acid secretion; used for treatment of duodenal ulcer

262. During the discharge planning session for a chronically ill infant, the nurse observes that the single mother nervously paces most of the time while bouncing the infant in her arms. Which of the following suggestions by the nurse is BEST?

1. "See your obstetrician for a prescription for a mild tranquilizer."
2. "Buy a commercially made 'baby bouncer' infant seat."
3. "Enroll in a Volunteers of America parenting class."
4. "Investigate hiring a live-in nanny."

Strategy: Answers are implementations. Determine the outcome of each answer choice. Is it desired?

(1) it is not the most beneficial action in the overall scope of the problem
(2) inappropriate to the situation
(3) *correct*—under these circumstances; will help both mother and baby
(4) parenting avoidance

263. The nurse is caring for clients on the postpartum unit. A client receiving heparin for the treatment of deep vein thrombosis (DVT) says to the nurse, "I am so upset that I can't breastfeed my infant." Which of the following statements, is made by the nurse, is BEST?

1. "You will be able to breastfeed your baby."
2. "Why do you think that it will be a problem?"
3. "We will check your baby's clotting times."
4. "We will give the baby protamine sulfate."

Strategy: Determine the outcome of each answer choice.

(1) *correct*—heparin not transmitted in breast milk; breastfeeding considered safe
(2) yes/no question, nontherapeutic
(3) heparin not transmitted to infant, only concerned about the mother's PTT
(4) is the antidote for heparin, not required

264. A client is experiencing a severe panic attack and has threatened to hurt another client on the unit. The nurse would expect to administer which of the following PRN medications as ordered?

1. Chlorpromazine (Thorazine).
2. Lithium carbonate (Lithane).
3. Haloperidol (Haldol).
4. Phenytoin (Dilantin).

Strategy: Think about the action of each medication.
(1) more likely to be used PRN when a client is experiencing agitation associated with schizophrenia
(2) an antimanic drug
(3) *correct*—Haldol is particularly effective in reducing assaultive behavior associated with severe anxiety
(4) an anticonvulsant medication

265. The nurse is caring for clients in the outpatient clinic. The nurse returns to the desk and is given four phone messages. Which of the following phone messages should the nurse return FIRST?

1. A client who has an indwelling Foley catheter and is complaining of foul-smelling urine.
2. A client who had a 9 lb infant 3 days ago and is complaining of painful breasts.
3. A client who had a cataract lens extraction 4 days ago and has not had a bowel movement in 3 days.
4. A client states that he had abdominal cramping and diarrhea after eating a large meal.

Strategy: Determine the least stable client.
(1) possible urinary tract infection (UTI) due to catheter; should force fluids, drink cranberry juice, antibiotics may be prescribed
(2) should encourage breastfeeding, not a priority
(3) *correct*—straining at stool increases intraocular pressure and should be avoided
(4) requires further investigation, not a priority

Coordinated Care

266. Which one of these tasks could be assigned to the certified nursing assistant?

A)   Feeding a client who has difficulty swallowing after a stroke

B)   Giving enemas until clear to a middle-aged man scheduled for a colonoscopy

C)   Performing a post-op dressing change

D)   Assisting a client with colostomy care 24 hours after surgery

The correct answer is B: Giving enemas until clear to a middle-aged man scheduled for a colonoscopy. The certified nursing assistant can be assigned tasks which have predictable outcomes.

267. The nursing student is discussing the delegation of tasks to an unlicensed assistive personnel (UAP) with a preceptor. Which task, assigned to the UAP by the student, indicates the student needs help with delegation?

A)   Assisting a client to ambulate

B)   Feeding a 2 year-old in traction

C)   Providing discharge teaching

D)   Collecting a sputum specimen

268. Which statement by the nurse is appropriate when asking an unlicensed assistive personnel (UAP) to assist a 69 year-old surgical client to ambulate for the first time?

A)   "Have the client sit on the side of the bed before starting to walk in the room."

B)   "If the client is dizzy on standing, ask the client to take some deep breaths."

C)   "Assist the client to the bathroom at least twice."

D)   "After you assist the client to the chair, let me know if any complaints of abnormal feelings by the client."

The correct answer is A: "Have the client sit on the side of the bed before starting to walk in the room.". Give clear information to the UAP about what is expected for client safety.

Infection Control

269. When a client is diagnosed with tuberculosis, the public health department is to be notified for what reason?

A)   Disease statistics need to be maintained

B)   Contacts need to be traced and screened

C)   The incidence of tuberculosis is on the rise

D)   Follow-up with additional tests are required

The correct answer is B: Contacts need to be traced and screened. Tuberculosis is a reportable disease because persons who had contact with the client must be traced, evaluated for the disease and possibly treated prophylactically.

270. A child has been admitted to the pediatric unit after swallowing a household cleaner. Which of these findings is more commonly associated with the fact that the poison was a corrosive?

A)   Burning mouth and throat pain

B)   Bradycardia and orthopnea

C)   Oliguria and cyanosis

D)   Diarrhea and vomiting

The correct answer is A: Burning mouth and throat pain. Local irritation of tissues is most closely associated with a corrosive poisoning.

271. Which of these actions is the first priority in the prevention of infections, whether in the hospital or home setting?

A)   Handwashing

B)   Use of antibacterial soaps

C)   Sneeze into the elbow with a bent arm

D)   Wash the hands before eating

The correct answer is A: Handwashing. Handwashing remains the most effective way to avoid spreading infection. However, too often nurses do not practice good handwashing techniques and do not teach families to do so. Nurses need to wash their hands before and after touching the client. Note that all of the options are correct actions to prevent infection. However the question asks for a priority.

Delegation of Care

272. A client is receiving an intravenous (IV) infusion via pump. When caring for this client, which one
of these actions can the nurse safely ask an unlicensed assistive personnel (UAP) to perform?

A)   Adjust the flow rate

B)   Monitor the pump's operation

C)   Change the IV dressing

D)   Report the reading on the pump for ml remaining

The correct answer is D: Report the reading on the pump for ml remaining. When directing the UAP, communicate clearly and specifically what the task is and what should be reported to the nurse. Only implementation or routine tasks should be assigned since routine tasks do not require independent judgment.

273. Which one of these clients would be most appropriate for a PN, who has been reassigned to a
different unit, to accept?

A)   A trauma victim with multiple lacerations requiring complex dressings

B)   An elderly client with cystitis and an indwelling urethral catheter

C)   A confused client whose family complains about the nursing care after surgery

D)   A client admitted for possible stroke with unstable neuro findings

The correct answer is B: An elderly client with cystitis and an indwelling urethral catheter. This is a stable client with predictable outcomes and no risk of instability.

274. The care of which of the following clients can be safely assigned to an unlicensed assistive personnel (UAP)?

A)   A client with peripheral vascular disease and an ulceration of the lower leg

B)   A pre-operative client awaiting adrenalectomy with a history of asthma

C)   An 82 year-old client with hypertension and self-reported non-compliance

D)   A new admission with a history of transient ischemic attacks and dizziness

The correct answer is A: A client with peripheral vascular disease and an ulceration of the lower leg. This client has a chronic condition and needs supportive care. The other clients would have outcomes that are not predictable.

Priority of Care

275. The partner of a client with Alzheimer's disease expresses concern about the burden of caregiving. Which action by the nurse should be a priority?

A)   Link the caregiver with a support group

B)   Suggest that friends need to visit regularly

C)   Schedule a home visit each week

D)   Develop a telephone support system

The correct answer is A: Link the caregiver with a support group. Assist caregivers to locate and join support groups. This is most helpful. Families share feelings and learn about services such as respite care. Health education is also available through local and national Alzheimer''s chapters.

276. The visiting nurse makes a postpartum home visit to a married female client. Upon arrival, the nurse observes that the client has a black eye and numerous bruises on her arms and legs. The next nursing intervention would be to

A)   Call the police to report indications of domestic violence

B)   Talk with the couple about the findings

C)   Leave the home because of the unsafe environment

D)   Interview the client without the partner to determine the origin of the injuries

The correct answer is D: Interview the client without the partner to determine the origin of the injuries. It would be wrong to assume domestic violence without further assessment. Separate the suspected victims from their partner until battering has been ruled out.

277. A client is admitted with severe injuries from an auto accident. The client's vital signs are BP 120/50, pulse rate 110, and respiratory rate of 28. The initial nursing intervention would be to

A)   Begin the ordered pain control therapy

B)   Initiate continuous blood pressure monitoring

C)   Administer oxygen therapy

D)   Institute cardiac monitoring

The correct answer is C: Administer oxygen therapy. Early findings of shock reveal hypoxia with rapid heart rate and respirations. Oxygen therapy is the most critical and the initial intervention. The other interventions are secondary to oxygen therapy and would occur in a sequence of options 4,2, and 1.

Nursing Care Management

278. Ms. T. is bedridden. The nurse is evaluating whether the family members understand how to position the client correctly. Which of the following should the nurse observe?

A) The extremities should always be extended to prevent contractures.

B) Lower arm and leg are always supported in the lateral positions.

C) The spine should have maximal lordosis in almost all positions.

D) The family should change the position at least every two hours.

The correct answer is D. Position changes should occur at least every two hours, more often if needed.

279. Ms. R. is bedridden and positioned on her right side. There is a pillow beneath her head. Her right
arm is extended near her hip. Her left leg is extended and parallel with the right leg. Which of the following is correct?

A) She should be semiprone with the weight on her upper chest.

B) Ms. O.'s right arm should be flexed at the shoulder and elbow.

C) There should not be a pillow under her head.

D) The client's right leg should be flexed at the hip and knee.

The correct answer is B. The lower arm should be flexed, so the body does not rest on it.

280. The nurse uses a wide stance when moving a heavy box of supplies. Which of the following is the best reason the nurse would do this? Because it

A) avoids back strain.

B) lowers the center of gravity.

C) increases stability.

D) contracts the muscles.

2The correct answer is C. The greater the stability, the less chance of injury. When increasing the
base of support, the nurse helps to maintain balance.

www.ingramcontent.com/pod-product-compliance
Lightning Source LLC
Chambersburg PA
CBHW051504170526
45166CB00001B/387